GW01373387

HOSPITAL SHIPS AND
AMBULANCE TRAINS

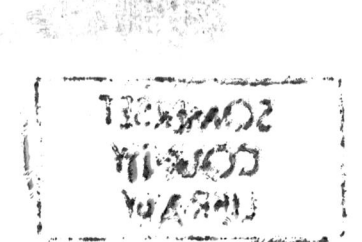

HOSPITAL SHIPS and AMBULANCE TRAINS

by
Lt-Colonel
John H. Plumridge
OBE, RAMC (Retd)

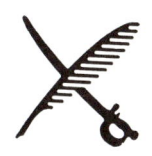

LONDON 1975
SEELEY, SERVICE & CO

First published in Great Britain 1975 by
SEELEY, SERVICE & CO. LTD.,
*196 Shaftesbury Avenue,
London WC2H 8JL*

Copyright © 1975 John H. Plumridge

ISBN 0 85422 087 9

Text set in 12 pt. Photon Imprint, printed by photolithography,
and bound in Great Britain at The Pitman Press, Bath.

*To
my wife*
*who has shared my interest in the
Corps—especially in ambulance
trains—since we met and married in
world war I and who has given me
invaluable help in the research
necessary for the writing of this book.*

CONTENTS

Acknowledgments 11
Foreword 12

1 Naval Hospital Ships Before 1918   13
2 Military Hospital Ships Before the First World War   21
3 Military Hospital Ships, Hospital Carriers and Ambulance Transports from 1914 to 1920   34
4 Naval and Military Hospital Ships and Carriers in the Second World War   51
5 The Naval Hospital Ship, HMHS *Maine*   67
6 Hospital Ships for Merchant Seamen and Deep-Sea Fishermen   72
7 The Beginning of Railway Ambulance Transport   80
8 Military Hospital Trains in the South African War   91
9 Military Ambulance Trains on Service Overseas in the First World War   98
10 Military Ambulance Trains in the United Kingdom in the First World War   125
11 Naval Ambulance Trains in the United Kingdom in the First World War   133
12 Military Ambulance Trains in the United Kingdom and Overseas in the Second World War   138
13 Casualty Evacuation Trains in the United Kingdom in the Second World War   149
14 Ambulance Trains and Hospital Ships Today and in the Future   156
15 Appreciation   160

APPENDICES

A	Naval Hospital Ships from 1608 to 1731	163
B	Hospital Ships on Service with the Royal Navy from 1790 to 1854	165
C	Military Hospital Ships and Ambulance Transports in the First World War	166
D	Hospital Ships and Other Vessels used for the Reception, Treatment and Movement of Casualties During the Gallipoli Campaign of 1915/1916	169
E	Naval and Military Hospital Ships and Carriers in the Second World War	170
F	Admissions of patients to Naval Hospital ships during the Second World War	172
G	The 'Princess Christian Hospital Train' in the South African War	173
H	No 4 Hospital Train in the South African War	174
J	Growth of the Military Ambulance Train Service in France in the Second World War	175
K	Capacity of Military Ambulance Trains in France, September 1915	177
L	First Battle of the Somme: Evacuation of casualties by Ambulance Train from 1 to 4 July, 1916	178
M	Description of No 63 American Ambulance Train for service in France in the First World War	181
N	Description of standard Ambulance Trains for service overseas in the First World War	183
O	Military Ambulance Trains in the United Kingdom in the First World War	185
P	Description of the War Department Ambulance Train—the 'Netley Coaches'	186
Q	No 1 Naval Ambulance Train in the United Kingdom in the First World War	187
	Bibliography	188

ILLUSTRATIONS

1. HMHS *Rewa* in Malta harbour (Imperial War Museum) — 19
2. The first Hospital Ship *Maine* (Imperial War Museum) — 32
3. Hospital Ship *Asturias* (Imperial War Museum) — 36
4. Hospital Ship *Loyalty* (RAMC Museum) — 37
5. The ward deck of the *Loyalty* (RAMC Museum) — 38
6. The *Aquitania* in the Mediterranean (Imperial War Museum) — 38
7. Hospital Ship *Britannic* (Imperial War Museum) — 39
8. Hospital Ship *Mauretania* (Imperial War Museum) — 40
9. River Hospital Ship *Nahba* (Imperial War Museum) — 41
10. The sinking of the *Anglia* (Imperial War Museum) — 43
11. The *Gloucester Castle* (Union Castle Line) — 45
12. Casualties at the Dardenelles (RAMC Museum) — 47
13. Stretcher cases at Boulogne (Imperial War Museum) — 49
14. Hospital Ship *Maid of Kent* (RAMC Museum) — 52
15. HMHS *Isle of Jersey* (RAMC Museum) — 53
16. Hospital Ship *St Julien* (RAMC Museum) — 53
17. The *Newfoundland* at Salerno (Imperial War Museum) — 55
18. Hospital Ship *Dinard* (RAMC Museum) — 56
19. HMHS *Vasna* (RAMC Museum) — 59
20. Hospital Ship *El Nil* (RAMC Museum) — 63
21. A converted ferry boat (Imperial War Museum) — 66
22. The fourth Hospital Ship *Maine* (Imperial War Museum) — 68

23 The last HMHS *Maine* (Imperial War Museum)	70
24 The railway works at Balaklava (*Illustrated London News*)	82
25 Cots ready for loading onto the Princess Christian Hospital Train	93
26 A ward car on the Princess Christian Hospital Train	94
27 One of the 'Netley Coaches' (Kate Pragnell)	95
28 The interior of a 'Netley Coach' (Kate Pragnell)	96
29 The Bréchot–Déspres–Amelines stretcher-carrying apparatus	99
30 The Bréchot apparatus folded for transport	100
31 King George V talking to patients (Imperial War Museum)	105
32 No 15 Princess Christian Hospital Train (Imperial War Museum)	112
33 No 23 British Ambulance Train (Imperial War Museum)	114
34 Walking wounded at Hinges (Imperial War Museum)	114
35 An overhead trolley in the trenches (Imperial War Museum)	115
36 The Barnton Tramway (Imperial War Museum)	117
37 Canadian wounded in horse-drawn trucks (Imperial War Museum)	118
38 Sitting wounded at Meteren (Imperial War Museum)	119
39 Repatriated German prisoners-of-war (Imperial War Museum)	123
40 RAMC staff entraining patients (Imperial War Museum)	126
41 No 63 Home Ambulance Train (A. G. Wells and Major F. A. Evans)	141
42 A ward coach on No 63 Home Ambulance Train (A. G. Wells and Major F. A. Evans)	142
43 No 33 Casualty Evacuation Train	150
44 No 33 coach in black-out conditions	151
45 The last ambulance train (Army Public Relations Office)	158

ACKNOWLEDGMENTS

I would like to express my particular thanks to the following who have helped me in this work. Mr M. Davies, Librarian, Royal Army College Library; Major-General A. MacLennan, OBE (Retd), Curator, Royal Army Medical Corps Historical Museum; Mr Martin Middlebrook, author of *First Day of the Somme;* The late Dame Beryl Oliver DBE RRC (Archivist) and Mrs C. F. Fawcett, both of the British Red Cross Society; Mr M. Sackett, HQ Southern Division, 1 Railway Group, Royal Corps of Transport; Colonel R. W. Scott, OBE (Retd) author of *Doctor to the Deep Sea Fisherman;* Mr D Tomlinson, Photographer, Royal Army Medical College; Major W. A. Winter, DCM (Retd), Regimental Headquarters, Royal Army Medical Corps. Also to the staffs of the British Transport Historical Records, the Imperial War Museum, the Public Record Office and of the Royal National Mission to Deep Sea Fishermen, the Treasurer, Seamen's Hospital Management Committee, the staffs of the Director-General, Army Medical Department and of the Medical Director to the Navy, both at the Ministry of Defence, the personnel of the Medical Directorate also the O.C. 79 Railway Squadron, Royal Corps of Transport, both of BAOR, the Medical Officer in Charge, Royal Naval Medical School, Alverstoke, Hants, the Librarians of the Royal Naval Medical Library, Haslar, Hants, and of the Naval Library, Empress State Buildings, London. I am also grateful to the following for permission to quote briefly from their publications. British Railways Eastern Region *Dunkirk and the Great Western* (Ashley Brown); British Railways London Midland Region *LMS at War* (C. C. Nash); William Blackmore and Sons Ltd *Diary of a Nursing Sister on the Western Front—1914/1915* (Sister K. E. Luard, RRC) and *The Rescue Ships* (Vice-Admiral H. B. Schofield and Lieut-Commander L. F. Martyn); Hodder and Stoughton *The Ships of Youth* (Geraldine Edge and Mary E. Johnston); Chatto and Windus Ltd *Unknown Warriors* (Sister K. E. Luard, RRC); The Director of Publishing, Her Majesty's Stationery Office *Official Histories of the Medical Services of the Second World War;* British Railways Southern Region *War on the Line—The Story of the Southern Railway in Wartime;* Cassell and Co Ltd *One Hundred Years of Army Nursing* (Ian Hay) and George C. Harrap and Co Ltd *Wilfred Grenfell—His Life and Work* (J. Lennox Kerr). Last but in no way least to all members of the staff of the Devon County Library, both at Exmouth and at Exeter who have given such friendly and continuous assistance.

I am also appreciative of the help of others too numerous to mention individually.

FOREWORD

The main aim of this book is to tell the story of the transport of the sick and wounded of the British armed forces by sea and rail—two forms of medical transport which are complementary to one another.

My particular interest is in ambulance trains, on which I did duty at home before and during the First World War, later in the war also serving overseas on them.

I cannot trace any other work devoted entirely to this subject, so I have taken my information from numerous assorted sources, including official and unofficial books and publications, documents, journals, newspapers, and other unexpected sources.

I hope the book will interest past and present members of the Medical Services of the Army (in which I served continuously, in the Royal Army Medical Corps, for nearly 42 years); it should similarly interest members of the Royal Naval Medical Service.

There will also be some appeal to the members of such voluntary organizations as the St John Ambulance Brigade, the British Red Cross Society and the St Andrew's Ambulance Association, who were so closely associated with these transport services.

Maybe it will also revive memories of numerous service and ex-service personnel, and of civilians who, as patients, travelled by these forms of ambulance transport.

Lastly I hope it will prove informative and interesting to the many railway enthusiasts in this country.

J. H. P.

CHAPTER 1

Naval Hospital Ships Before 1918

It is impossible to say when a navy first used a vessel specifically as a hospital ship, though there is an allegation that the Spanish Armada fleet in 1587–1588 included fifteen of them. There is, however, considerable detailed information on hospital ships in the Royal Navy from as early as 1608. Dr J. J. Sutherland's article in the October, 1936, issue of *The Mariner's Mirror*—'The Hospital Ship 1608–1740' —provided invaluable information, as well as a definition of early hospital ships which is no less adequate today: 'a vessel equipped primarily to receive sick and wounded sailors, to provide them with interim treatment, and to convey them to hospitals or lodging houses on shore'. (At this point it is worthwhile to point out the difference between naval and military hospital ships. Naval hospital ships form a permanent part of the fleet—in the Royal Navy they are called Her Majesty's Hospital Ship, abbreviated as HMHS—while military hospital ships are brought into use only when occasion demands.)

Apart from their almost proven use in the French and Spanish fleets, the English Navy was the main user of hospital ships in the seventeenth century, Sweden, Denmark, Germany and the United Provinces depending solely on provisions made on board individual vessels. England's first recorded hospital ship was the *Goodwill* in 1608, and two accompanied a West Indies expedition in 1654. These, however, were special cases and it was not until after the Restoration in 1660 that the Navy made a regular practice of setting aside particular ships for hospital use.

Before that, Naval surgeons and mates were among the complement of all large ships; while a first rate ship of 800 men might not have had sick berth facilities, she would have had a medical crew of up to ten. Medical crews—all treated as seamen rather than as officers—were later allocated to most ships, the size of the crew depending on the type, armament and tonnage of the ship. Thus, while practically every vessel had a surgeon, there were no mates on cutters of 8 or 12 guns, though sloops and frigates (30–50 guns) had two mates. Surgeons on ships of the line (60–80 guns) were provided with three mates, and with five on the three-decker first and second rate ships (90–130 guns).

Throughout the reigns of Charles II and James II 'old sixth rates or hired merchantmen' were commissioned as hospital ships, though no more than two were ever in use simultaneously. They were 'made more commodious by cutting ventilation gratings in the sides' and the medical staff generally comprised a surgeon, four surgeon's mates and three attendants.

In the war against France in 1689 at first the usual two hospital ships were commissioned, but this rose to four in 1691, five in 1693 and to six in 1696. In Queen Anne's reign (1702–1714) this earlier experience caused six hospital ships to be put into service shortly after the declaration of hostilities. In 1703 the medical staff of hospital ships was increased by the addition of nurses and laundresses, who were paid at the rate of ordinary seamen. Two years later there were five nurses and three laundresses in addition to eight assistants on each hospital ship. Sailors' wives apparently served on hospital ships in the early stages of Anne's reign, but 'their predilection for drink led to their replacement by male nurses'. Between 1707 and 1711 there was an allocation of 300 beds (and 550 sheets) to the hospital ships *Martha* and *Leake*—compared with the 'two or three douzen bedds ruggs and pillows' and 'about twenty pairs of ould sheets' allowed in the 1665–1667 inventories.

By 1730 the recognized practice of converting vessels for use as hospital ships was 'to flush the gun deck, removing cabins and bulkheads; to separate off infectious cases flimsy deal or canvas partitions were used; two pairs of sheets were allowed to each bed'. The staff then frequently consisted of the surgeon, his assistant, four mates, a baker and four laundresses. There is also a reference in Dr Sutherland's article to surgeons who served on the *Ossory* and the *Orford* but neither of these vessels is included in the list of 34 hospital ships in service with the navy during the years 1608–1740. Practically all were 'gunships' varying from 78 to 664 tons, and with crews numbering from 30 to 95.

In the April, 1937, issue of *The Mariner's Mirror* Pierre Le Conte referred to Dr Sutherland's article on hospital ships and stated that most French fleets of the seventeenth century were accompanied by hospital ships (usually a storeship) but sometimes prizes or merchantmen; as a rule they were specially equipped and were called *flûte hôpital* or *hôpital de l'armée*. He appended an incomplete list of such vessels and named *La Fortune* (1639), *Le Saint-Jacques de Portugal* (1648), *La Flûte Royale*, wrecked on the coast of Corsica when acting as a hospital ship (1665), *Le Grand Saint-Augustin* (1666) and *Le Bien Chargé* (1673).

Other sources of information refer to early efforts to ameliorate the condition of sick and wounded English sailors. The 'Sick and Wounded (or Sick and Hurt) Board' was established in 1653, the duties of the Commissioner requiring his attendance at the nearest port after an action where he rented sick quarters and hired nurses and surgeons. It was in the same year during the Dutch Wars that naval ships were allowed medical comforts to the value of £5 per 100 men for each six months.

There also appears to have been a 'Florence Nightingale' of this period—one Elizabeth Alkin, commonly called 'Parliament Joan' because she nursed the wounded during the Civil War. On the outbreak of the Dutch Wars she volunteered for nursing service among the sailors at Portsmouth and later went on similar duty to Harwich.

Apart from temporary hospitals at places such as Deal there were no established naval hospitals in England and beds for sick and wounded sailors were requisitioned at Bart's and St Thomas's, while the derelict Savoy and Ely hospitals in London were also requisitioned.

There are many records of naval hospital ships in the last decade of the eighteenth century. HMS *Tournelle* was used as a hospital hulk at Bermuda while HMS *Pharon* did hospital ship duty on the 'Glorious First of June'. On 5 May, 1793, a fleet of 39 vessels, 26 of which were sail of the line, included a hospital ship, while the *Charon* served in that capacity on 23 June, 1795, when Lord Bridport's fleet of 29 vessels was in action. (The *Charon* was rated as a '44 gun vessel'.) In 1797 HMS *Argonaut* was the base hospital at Chatham, at which port she remained until 1828. HMS *Gorgon* was employed as a hospital ship in the 1814 American War, while on 1 January, 1826, a Charles Elliot RN was acting Commander on the *Seraphis* —described as a 'convalescent ship' at Port Royal, Jamaica. On 14 April at Port Royal he was confirmed in his appointment to the *Magnificent* which is stated to have been a 'hospital and store ship'.

During the China War of 1839–1842 HMS *Minden* was the hospital ship for the fleet and in 1854 naval vessels sailed to the Crimea loaded with stores and returned to England with sick and wounded naval personnel. Hospital muster books which cover the period 1793–1854 record the names of twenty-nine vessels employed by the navy as hospital ships (see Appendix B).

The first naval hospital ship with any appreciable length of service appears to be the 90-gun HMS *Victor Emanuel*, which was launched in 1855 and converted into a hospital ship during the Ashanti War of 1873–1874. HMS *Simon* was similarly used in that war while HMS *Coromandel* was a hospital ship in the later Ashanti War of 1878. (It is not clear, however, whether these vessels were naval or military hospital ships.) HMS *Coromandel* again did hospital ship duty in the West African campaigns in 1895 and HMS *Malcolm* served as a naval hospital ship two years later.

Up until the First World War fully equipped hospital ships kept with the Fleet as long as they could; after engagements sailors were taken aboard for return to port and base hospital, though frequently those ships that were returning to port kept their wounded in their own sick bays until they recovered or could be transferred direct to the base hospital. (In peacetime, the base hospital itself would frequently be one of the hospital ships.)

The situation changed considerably during the Great War, however. The large number of casualties led to overcrowding and this made the ships unsuitable as base hospitals. Instead they became casualty clearing stations, receiving and treating patients, and transferring the more serious cases to shore bases. The greater mobility of vessels by 1914 also meant they were able to return to port more frequently—something they had to do often in order to refuel. Hospital ships in the First World War therefore stopped accompanying the Fleet on patrol or into battle areas, but remained nearby or in deep water ports.

On the outbreak of the First World War the Admiralty ordered the conversion of three ocean-going liners into naval hospital ships and another six vessels were taken over as the war progressed. They were equipped with from 200 to 300 beds and most of them were made ready for sea in about three weeks. Among the naval hospital ships which saw service in the war were the *Agadir, Asturias, Cecelia, China, Classic, Drina, Garth Castle, Guildford Castle, Karapara, Ophir, Oxfordshire, Plassy, Rewa, St Margeret of Scotland, Salta, Somali* and *Soudan*. The *St Margaret of Scotland,* formerly the *Balentia,* was provided and equipped for the navy by the Scottish Branch of the British Red Cross Society. All the staff were Scotsmen and the £20,000 raised by flag-days and other activities also provided twelve ambulance motor-launches for use in the Dardanelles, Egypt and Salonika.

Many of the later naval hospital ships had accommodation in excess of 300 beds, but HMHS *Drina* was typical of the smaller ships. She accommodated 221 patients in many wards, one of which had 16 beds for officers, while a smaller one had four beds for warrant officers. Six wards of varying capacity from 21 to 46 beds were used for ratings, and an eight-bedded ward for infectious cases; mental patients were segregated in a small three-bedded ward. The *Drina* carried a Senior Medical officer and six surgeons, a dental officer, a chaplain, four nursing sisters, 16 Royal Naval Sick Berth staff and 32 auxiliaries of that staff. In spite of her 221 beds, her greatest load once totalled 900 patients.

Naval hospital ships did duty at the Gallipoli beaches during the Dardanelles campaign, one being HMHS *Soudan,* which had been converted from a transport of 6,700 tons and had accommodation for 202 patients—taking over 300 in an emergency. During the first operations, between 25 February and 19 March, 1915, she took on a total of 137 naval casualties. The next operations, from 25 April to 1 May, again saw her on service in that area. On the first day a destroyer came alongside with two dead and five wounded; by evening, however, 352 army casualties had been embarked; then 25 naval casualties were admitted. Later, when the patients totalled 420, HMHS *Soudan* drew off so that the wounded could be more carefully and efficiently treated. On 27 April all the military cases were transferred to the army hospital carrier *Argon* which was bound for Alexandria. This left the *Soudan* with 70 cases, but on 29 April a further 38 were received. Her next move was to Gaba Tepe where 83 cases were transferred to the hospital carrier *Somali* for passage home to the United Kingdom. The more seriously wounded were retained and yet further casualties were embarked on the first two days of May. Then the *Soudan* moved off to a safer anchorage, 733 casualties having been treated on the ship since 25 February. On 17 May she again went to Gaba Tepe and took on 328 casualties from the Australian and New Zealand contingents, later transferring 102 of the less seriously wounded to the hospital carrier *Galeka*. During 20 and 21 May 97 more wounded were taken on board and on the latter day HMHS *Soudan* at last left the Dardanelles. She reached Malta three days later when all army patients were transferred to the Military Hospital, Valetta.

HMHS *Rewa* began her duties on 29 January, 1915, and left Gallipoli with her last load of patients on 29 April bound for England. During this period 7,424 patients were taken on board, of whom 3,647 were discharged to the advance base; 3,628 were taken by the ship to naval hospitals at Malta, Alexandria and Plymouth, but 149 patients died on board. Subsequently HMHS *Rewa*—although illuminated as a hospital ship—was torpedoed on 4 January, 1918, a few miles south-west of Lundy Island approaching the Bristol channel. The explosion killed four of the engine-room crew and

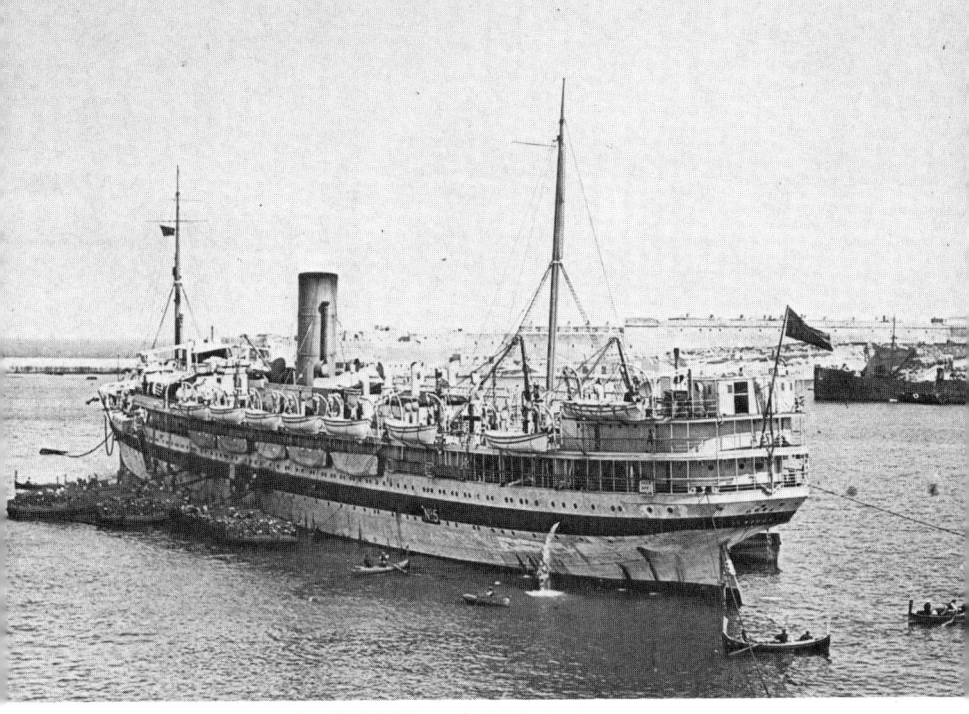

1 HMHS *Rewa* in Malta harbour

shattered two life-boats. The ship was full of cot and walking-patients at the time but nearby vessels—two drifters and the *Paul Paix*—took all of them on board and landed them at Swansea the following day.

Two private yachts were hired by the Navy for hospital ship duty. The *Grianaig* was taken over in 1916 but was subsequently used by the Army from 4 July, 1918, until February, 1919, when she was returned to her owners. The *Liberty* was used as a naval hospital ship from 1915 to January, 1919.

In the Battle of Jutland on 2 June, 1916, hospital boats were used to collect casualties from the fighting ships and transfer them to the naval hospital ships anchored in the Firth of Forth, the casualties from HMS *Princess Royal* being embarked on HMHS *Plassy*. Another, smaller hospital ship, HMHS *China*, was also in the area, while among the naval hospital ships which were at Scapa Flow during the First World War were HMHS *Classic* and HMHS *Karapara*.

A different, but very important vessel at Scapa Flow was the *Flying Kestrel*—a stout sea-going tug which was a 'fetch and carry' vessel servicing the British Fleet at Scapa Flow practically throughout the War. During her normal duties she delivered nearly a quarter of a million tons of fresh water, 60,000 bags of mail, and 2,000 tons of ammunition, rations and supplies. She also ferried about 25,000 men to and from Scrabster. In between these 'maid-of-all-work' duties she made a score or so rescues—on one occasion taking off the crew of 54 from the collier *Harmonic* under the most hazardous circumstances. Her importance as far as this book is concerned is that when vessels came in with casualties it was the *Flying Kestrel* which took the stretcher cases to Scrabster, on their way to a base hospital.

The military hospital ship *Panama* which had been used by the army in the First World War was taken over by the Navy in 1920 and renamed HMHS *Maine*. Her eventful story appears later.

CHAPTER 2

Military Hospital Ships Before the First World War

The principal function of military hospital ships is to carry an active army's sick and wounded from overseas bases to home ports, where ambulance trains distribute the casualties to hospitals throughout the country. Both sea and rail medical transport services are thus closely linked, but since ships have been in existence for so long, it is impossible to say when a vessel was first used for such hospital purposes. One early reference, however, is of a hospital ship being included in an expeditionary force sent to the West Indies during Oliver Cromwell's brief rule in the seventeenth century; and there is a French claim to a similar use of sea-going vessels in that century.

The first documented record of specific English ships being used as hospital ships comes from the reign of Charles II, when on 29 August, 1683, a fleet of 29 vessels 'including nine warships' sailed for Tangier. Two—the *Unity* and the *Welcome* had been fitted out as hospital ships. On the evacuation of Tangier the *Unity* sailed in October with 114 invalid soldiers and 104 women and children. During the next month the *Welcome* took off another batch of sick soldiers and families, and female nurses were aboard both vessels to care for the patients.

Then in 1714 hospital ships again accompanied an expedition—this time to Cartagena. It appears, however, that they were without surgeons, nurses or even cooks, and the accommodation and facilities were extremely poor. It was recorded, for instance, that the patients were driven to washing their wounds with their brandy ration!

On the withdrawal of troops from Willemstad in January, 1749, two vessels were used as hospital ships—the *Jean* and the *Herring*. The former took 69 patients to Ipswich, while the *Herring* sailed to London carrying 'the sick men of the Guards with lingering distempers—being 89 in number'.

It was not until 1800, however, that the question of the use of hospital ships for the army received serious consideration and on 2 July of that year T. Keate (Surgeon-General in the army) submitted 'to the consideration of His Royal Highness the Commander in Chief, and the Secretary at War, some remarks on Hospital Ships with a view to elucidating the utility of obtaining 44 gun ships of war for that service'. His letter pointed out that on the embarkation of troops for service abroad 'every space which can afford a berth for a soldier is taken up ... leaving no part of the vessel suitable to the reception of Sick Men, excepting such whose indisposition is too trifling to require segregation'. He argued that 'a distinct vessel or two for the reception of Men with diseases of a contagious or a dangerous tendency' would greatly relieve the transports which built up a large proportion of sick.

Surgeon-General Keate noted that 'such vessels should be in readiness and properly appointed to receive the Wounded of an Army taking the Field and more particularly in invading an enemy country where houses or hospitals are seldom to be provided in time'.

He made mention of the fact that 'The late service in Holland is a case in point, for without the *Asia,* which is acknowledged to be one of the best hospital ships that has ever been employed, the whole of the Wounded Men on the first day of the Action must have inevitably been left on the Beach for at least 24 hours, by which many more lives would have been lost'. Keate went on to emphasize that vessels should be held in readiness 'to convey home such Sick or Wounded as require a change of climate, or which from their numbers embarrass the Hospitals on Service and therefore ought to be sent away for their relief.

Not surprisingly, Keate criticized the conditions in some ships, emphasizing the necessity for cleanliness and pointing out that poor ventilation increased the chances of contagious diseases spreading throughout the ships. No vessel was ever built to be a hospital ship, and little reconstruction was done on designated ships. Keate recorded that they were usually 'common Transports with few or no Ports, very low between Decks'. Their method of construction, with beams and spars in abundance, made it very difficult to maintain cleanliness, and on top of that 'the Masters ... for unanswerable reason object to additional ports being opened on the sides'. The only ventilation in the ships designed to carry merchandise came from deck openings, which apparently was not very efficient. Keate suggested that merchant ships should not be used any more and wrote that 'I have been induced to propose Ships of War, or the East Indiamen, to be substituted for that service'.

A visit by Keate to Deptford to inspect ships recommended to be used as hospital ships disclosed that only one—the *Niger*—seemed suitable, being 'tolerably airy and accommodating about 50 men'. She was 'rather too low between Decks, though deeper than the *Lady Juliana* ... and in every respect better than this ill contrived Vessel'. The Surgeon-General recommended 'this Vessel be taken into the Service and that two or three more of a similar or larger description may be engaged as permanent Vessels so as to have Hospital Ships always in readiness'.

Then he stressed the need for more ample and frequent means of bringing invalids home from the West Indies by saying that 'many of the Men with ulcers and most of those with incipient chronic diseases, if sent to Europe in time, would be completely restored to health and such as would not be perfectly recovered might still be employed in Garrisons at Home'.

Keate's letter went on to suggest the allocation of two hospital ships each for the Leeward Islands and for Jamaica, raising the point that on their outward journeys they could carry out the troops and stores which always had to get there somehow. The supposed immunity for hospital ships against attack was not even considered at that time, and Keate suggested that if the vessels were armed they would not need an escort home. The growth of westward trade also prompted the opinion that a small hospital at Falmouth would benefit ships returning from the West Indies, which would then not have to carry on to Gosport or Plymouth. The letter ended with the writer saying that 'Hospital Ships ought to have at least 450 tonnage with between 7 and 8 feet depth between decks, and five or six large ports of a side'.

A second letter on the same subject was dated 15 December, 1806. It was written by a regimental officer, Lieutenant-Colonel J. H. Gordon, and it again referred to Jamaica and to 'sore legs'. It transmitted a Report of the Medical Board of Health held on 28 May, 1806, on the same subject. His views, which were at variance with those expressed by the Medical Board of Health, were, however, supported by Joshua Rocket, then in the army medical department and holding the appointment of Deputy Inspector of Hospitals, West Indies.

Colonel Gordon's letter is interesting because it refers to hospital ships out of the context of transporting the wounded, and compares their merits directly with 'wooden hospitals on shore'. The extreme heat in Jamaica afflicted his regiment, and doubtless a well-ventilated ship could have been more bearable. The 'sore legs . . . condition' also resulted in a point in favour of hospital ships, for the malady 'increased with astonishing rapidity as to bafflle every mode of cure but sea air'. Something else which took its toll, though with the victim's acquiescence, was the 'easy access to Rum on the Island'. The fact that 'Rum would not be readily available to patients on board ships' helped decide Gordon in favour of hospital ships against shore hospitals as much as did the advantage of changing its moorings 'from time to time as circumstances . . . might render necessary'.

A few years later consideration was given to the need for hospital ships during the Peninsular War (1808–1814) and it was also proposed that they should accompany the expedition sent to Walcheren in Holland. The outcome of this latter proposal was not recorded but it is known that in the force of 39,000 troops there were 23,000 deaths in four months. Some use of hospital sea-transport was made during the Peninsular War, however; an order from the Adjutant-General's office at Busaco of 22 September, 1810, said 'The sick of the 3rd Division will find boats at Pena Cova to transport them to Coimbra'. The patients were ordered to 'carry two days provisions ready cooked'.

There is one reference from 1815 to the use of water transport for patients which states that 'canal boats carried wounded to hospital after the battle of Waterloo'. Then there followed a lull of almost four decades before the question of military hospital ships was seriously raised once more—on the outbreak of the Crimean War.

In May, 1854, Andrew Smith, the Director General of the Army and Ordnance Medical Departments, planned the provision of hospital ships and took into account not only the transport of patients but their reception and treatment as well. His plans were ignored by the military authorities and it became necessary for both sail and steam transports to be adapted for the evacuation of sick and wounded—to the detriment of the patients—and in the following month the War Minister ordered the naval authorities to ask the Turkish Government to provide a line-of-battle ship for use as a floating hospital.

In July Inspector General John Hall, the Principal Medical Officer of the Crimean Force, urged the necessity of having steamers set aside and fitted up as hospital ships. As a result the *Andes* and the *Cambria* (reported at the time as 'ill-calculated for such use') were provided by the naval authorities at Varna where the British Army was concentrating. Surgeons, regimental orderlies and medical stores were put on board and the two vessels then carried wounded after the Battle of Alma (20 September, 1854) from the Crimea to Scutari—a journey of about 300 miles across the Black Sea. Some of the casualties from this battle were also evacuated to a hospital at Cadkciry which was just beyond the barracks at Scutari. When convalescent they were transferred to an old 'two-decker Turkish Hulk' which for years had been rotting at Kassim Point, and which had been converted for hospital use and anchored off Seraglio.

In the meantime, on 11 August, 1854, Hall wrote to the Quartermaster General saying that in the event of the British Army embarking in force from Varna, conveyance was required for at least 400 tons of medical and purveyors stores besides the men, wagons and horses of the 'ambulance-train'.

He emphasized that it would be especially convenient for the whole to be shipped on board vessels that 'were to be used as hospital ships'. In September, two other ships—the *Bombay* (a wooden paddle steamer) and the *Mercia*—were also taken into use for the movement of patients from Varna to Scutari.

Then came the outbreak of cholera at Varna, and to cope with this Staff Surgeon Angus Mackay and Assistant Surgeon James Wishart were put in medical charge of the steamship *Kangaroo* while Assistant Surgeon Henry Sylvester embarked on the sailing ship *Dunbar*. These two ships, with their complement of patients, made the journey to Scutari together—the *Kangaroo* towing the sailing vessel.

Also in September the *Avon* carried 340 wounded Russian prisoners-of-war to Odessa under the care of Assistant Surgeon James Thomson, who was the Regimental Surgeon of the 44th (the East Essex) Regiment of Foot. Surgeon Thomson was with his regiment at the Battle of Alma and had volunteered to remain behind with about 700 desperately wounded Russians after the British troops had been withdrawn. Although he was alone, he was able to restore almost half the Russian wounded to a reasonable state of health and then take them to Odessa. Unfortunately the strain and the privation he endured resulted in his death on 5 October, 1854; but his courageous conduct was later 'noticed in both Houses of Parliament'.

Subsequently the *Avon* became the first vessel told off by the Agents of Transports for the reception of sick and wounded and to be specially inspected by the medical authorities for that purpose. The inspection was carried out by Staff Surgeon Major Tice, the Principal Medical Officer at Balaklava. His report on 17 November to Inspector General Hall stated: '*Avon*, 1,400 tons, 6 ft 6 inches between decks. On board *Avon* 25 beds, 1,200 blankets or thereabouts, 700 pounds of tea, 6 hundredweight of sugar—Government property. Medical comforts to be had on board on requisition as follows—rice, sago, arrowroot, essence of beef, boiled beef—private property and all of a liberal supply. The *Avon* to be furnished with as little delay as possible in the usual proportion for 350.' On the following day she began embarking 311 British patients and on 4 December left for Scutari.

On 25 November the *Trent* carried a further 185 invalids from Balaklava to Scutari, being followed on 11 December by the *Sydney*. Also in 1854 the *Pride of the Ocean*—a large transport which had been damaged in a hurricane—was converted into a hulk for the reception of patients. During the spring of 1855 another four vessels—the *Orient, St Hilda, Robert Sale* and *William Jackson*—were converted to accommodate 100 patients each.

Generally all these so-called hospital ships were loaded with sick and wounded far in excess of their capacity and the plight of the patients during the voyage across the Black Sea from Crimea to Scutari was often deplorable. The surgeons who were detailed to look after the patients did their best—but at that time there were no nurses, and the Army Hospital Corps had yet to be formed so there were no trained orderlies either. The few regimental orderlies on the ships did all they could, but many were themselves unfit or very old.

In April, 1855, two hospital ships—probably the *Saladin* and the *Great Tasmania,* which had fixed berths for 400 and 570 patients respectively—were taken into service. Each had a permanent staff of one surgeon, two assistant surgeons, as well as wardmasters, stewards and orderlies, some of whom subsequently became members of the 'Corps of Hospital Orderlies' then under consideration. Rules for the running of these hospital ships were published in May, and it was during this month that it was decided to regularize the use of regimental orderlies on board ships and that 'strong inducements should be held out to men who would take upon themselves the duties of hospital orderlies on board transports'. An instruction of 5 May, 1855, which specifically referred to the *Saladin* and the *Great Tasmania* as hospital ships, gave details of the method of selection of such personnel, their duties, ranks and the numbers to be provided for each of the two vessels; and of the most important inducement of all (especially when volunteers are being called for) their rates of pay. Each vessel was to have a steward with the rank of sergeant-major and paid 5/- a day; there was to be one wardmaster ranking as a colour-sergeant and another as a corporal but both on the same daily rate of pay at 2/6d; and 25 orderlies for the *Saladin* and 40 for the *Great*

Tasmania—all privates and drawing pay at 2/– a day. Those who were entitled to good conduct pay continued to receive it at the rates and under the conditions then in force, and volunteers were taken from men deemed by medical officers to be 'unfit to proceed on service'.

An additional and most important inducement was that they could eventually obtain admission to the proposed 'Corps of Hospital Orderlies' and that their service in that Corps would count from the date on which they were accepted for duty on the hospital ships. (The Corps, which was formed on 11 June, 1855, was actually called the 'Medical Staff Corps'. It was replaced by the 'Army Hospital Corps' on 1 August, 1857, reverted to its original title on 20 September, 1884, and finally became the Royal Army Medical Corps on 23 June, 1898.)

During the last three months of 1854, 41 vessels of one kind or another carried 8,106 sick and wounded from the Crimea to Scutari—516 of whom died on board. In the first three months of 1855 36 vessels evacuated 6,380 cases to hospitals in the Bosphorus but the number who died during the voyages is unknown. In addition to the nearly 14,500 British patients, 202 wounded Russian prisoners were taken to Scutari during this period. Some of the casualties from the Battle of Inkerman on 5 November, 1854, had been taken to Malta, and during the whole of the Crimean War (April, 1854 to July, 1856) altogether 11,500 sick and wounded were invalided home to Britain.

The first occasion when vessels were specifically equipped and fitted out as 'floating hospitals' to attend an army on active service was during the China operations of 1860. The *Melbourne* and the *Mauritius,* both sail-rigged steam ships of over 2,000 tons, were adapted under the supervision of the Director General and other officers of the Army Medical Department. The *Melbourne* sailed for China on 13 January and the *Mauritius* four days later, each with a staff of five surgeons and 20 members of the newly formed Medical Staff Corps. Later, two wooden transports were similarly fitted up in China. The whole of the lower decks, where there was approximately 8 ft between decks, was used for hospital purposes, and each of the 125 patients had an allotment of some 230 cubic feet. Berths were provided and each had a small tray suspended above, which the patient could raise or lower, while a rope handle could be used to help him change his position in his bed. Personal belongings were stored in a small rack under each berth.

Wooden enclosures were added to the fore part of the main deck to shelter convalescents and separate cabins were provided for officer patients. There were adequate bathing and toilet arrangements and facilities for washing and drying clothes and linen. Particular attention was at last given to ventilation of the wards, and when bad weather kept the port-holes closed a large number of the most up-to-date ventilators led from numerous points to the upper deck. Another welcome innovation was the inclusion of 'Stevens' Dough-Mixing Machines' to ensure a continuous supply of fresh bread.

The surgery was in the centre of the ship and was immediately beneath a sky-light which provided light not only for the surgeons but also for dispensing medicines. The top of the sky-light was moveable, permitting patients to be placed on the operating table direct from the main deck. Together, the surgery and the dispensary formed a most extensive section. Two sides and one end were fitted with shelves holding over 200 bottles of 'lotions and potions'; all poisonous substances were contained in Messrs Savory and Moore's 'patent safeguard bottles'.

Another early reference to the movement of invalids by sea was in the mid 1860s when sailing transports were hired and specially fitted for the repatriation of invalid British troops from India to the United Kingdom. At that time these vessels were regarded as 'hospital ships' and in 1865 they brought home over 3,000 patients from India. All came from the Presidency ports—1,639 from Bengal, 539 from Bombay and 900 from Madras. On arrival in the United Kingdom the patients went to the Royal Victoria Hospital, Netley.

From 1865 there is also a reference to a 'floating hospital' being used on the Mississippi River.

In the Turco-Servian War of 1876 a British Red Cross Society mission provided a hospital barge with 25 beds on a covered deck and a further 25 below for the conveyance of sick and wounded from Semendria (Smederevo) and other Danube towns to Belgrade. This barge was towed by steamers passing up and down the Danube.

The SS *Ganges,* a new steel-hulled ship, was fitted out as a hospital ship for the Suakin expedition of 1885. She had wards on separate decks and also provided special accommodation for mental and for convalescent patients.

In the Russo-Turkish War of 1877–1878 the British Red Cross Society bore the cost of chartering and equipping the *Belle of Dunkerque* as a hospital ship. She sailed on 11 June, 1887, with Mr J. S. Young, Chief Commissioner, and five surgeons. She carried a cargo (valued at £7,000) which included drugs such as quinine and morphia, and also carbolic acid and chloroform. There were also numerous other items of medical equipment which would be practically unobtainable in the regions of the Black Sea. Constantinople was reached early in July and the ship then went on to Trebizond and Batum and eventually to Suchum Kaleh, where between 60 and 70 patients—together with doctors and attendants—were embarked on 1 August. The voyage was completed on 8 September and the patients were then transferred to what had been the barrack hospital at Scutari. Later in the month the *Belle of Dunkerque* was employed in carrying the sick and wounded to Constantinople and in distributing instruments and supplies to medical units in the area. There is also a reference that in this war the *Osmanieh* with a surgeon in charge made a trip with about 300 patients.

In 1882 a British expedition went to Egypt for the suppression of the Arabi revolt and some of the nursing sisters sent out by the War Office are stated to have been employed on hospital ships, probably the *Carthage* and *Courland.*

In the Egyptian Campaign of 1884–1885 the British Red Cross Society again gave assistance—this time for the comfort and welfare of British casualties. In January, 1885, the Society presented the steam launch *Queen Victoria,* this being the first time it provided a complete, self-contained unit to supplement army medical establishments in wartime. The vessel, under the charge of Dr White, plied the Nile between Cairo and Wadi Halfa—a distance of 800 miles. Wadi Halfa was first reached on 3 February, the *Queen Victoria* carrying medical stores for the hospitals on the upstream journeys. On the return journeys to Cairo invalids were carried on board, as well as in *dahabeahs,* which were towed behind. Three other vessels were used for the movement of sick and wounded in this campaign—the hospital ship *Ganges,* the steam launch *Princess* and the yacht *Stella.* The *Princess* towed horse-boats which had been adapted to carry patients while the *Stella* evacuated patients from Suakin. There is also a reference that the SS *Lileham* was used for hospital ship duties in this campaign. The stern-wheel steamer *Alexandra* also saw service with this expedition—again at the expense of the British Red Cross Society. She was constructed at Glasgow, transported in sections to Alexandria and eventually assembled at Cairo in June, 1885. Built to carry 48 patients, she did service on the lower reaches of the Nile between Assuan and Assiut. On the termination of hostilities she was presented to the British Government for use by the Army Medical Authorities.

In June, 1898, an expedition was sent to the Sudan and the British Red Cross Society again gave help. By 13 September the *Mayflower* had been chartered and converted to carry 52 patients under normal conditions and up to 72 in an emergency. Under command of Lieutenant N. H. Ross RAMC, she embarked her first patients at Assuan. Nursing sisters Isabella Gibson, Elizabeth Geddes and Anna Burke—all of the National Society for Aid to Sick and Wounded in time of war—did duty on the boat. In addition there were eight NCOs and men of the newly formed Royal Army Medical Corps. This was the first occasion on which the British Red Cross Society and the Army Medical Services worked together as one unit—thus forging an enduring link between the Society and the Army.

In the Spanish-American War of 1898 the United States Government fitted out six hospital ships—some of which were permanently attached to the fleet. In addition to the *Missouri* (sister ship of the *Maine* used by the British in the South African War) were the *Bay State, Relief* and *Solace.*

In the South African War of 1899–1902 transports were requisitioned and specially fitted out to accommodate and carry the sick and wounded. Two, the *Spartan* and the *Trojan,*

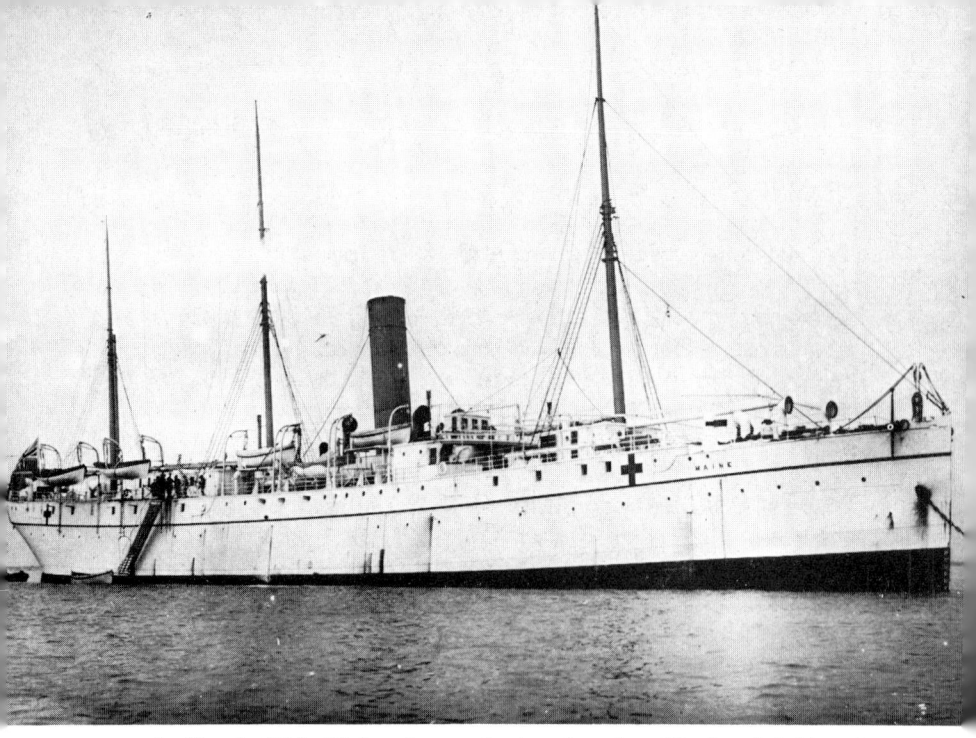

2 Hospital Ship *Maine*: she was the first of a series of five hospital ships of that name which served with the Navy from 1920 to 1954

had been launched in 1880 and 1881. The *Spartan* was requisitioned at Southampton in October, 1899, and converted into a hospital ship. Much of her service in this capacity was the movement of sick and wounded from Durban to the base hospitals at Cape Town. Her sister ship, the *Trojan,* similarly requisitioned and converted, was said to be the second vessel in the world to have electric light—a single lamp in the saloon!

The *Egypt* and the *Orcana* were converted at Durban to transfer patients to England. Another, the *German,* embarked the first trainload of patients from the Princess Christian Hospital Train. In addition there was the *Maine* which was converted into a hospital ship by a Committee of American Ladies in London under the Presidency of Lady Randolph Churchill. The story of this ship continues in a later chapter.

Lastly there was the *Princess of Wales* which was formerly the yachting cruiser *Midnight Sun.* She was fitted out as a hospital ship by the Central Committee of the Red Cross from funds remaining after the Suez Campaign of 1885—this money being made available by the Princess of Wales herself, who took a special interest in the vessel. This hospital ship accommodated 200 patients and made three voyages between Cape Town and England. She also carried patients between Cape Town and Durban, where, in addition, she acted as a stationary hospital ship outside the port.

The hospital ship *Maine* was used with other hospital ships, including the *Gwalior,* during the Boxer Rebellion of 1900, and the *Hardinge* was employed during the Somaliland operations of 1902–1904.

A number of military hospital ships were used by both sides in the Russo-Japanese war of 1904, and the British ship *Nubia* was a peacetime hospital ship in that year.

In the Turko-Balkan War of 1912–1913 an unnamed hospital ship was employed at Salonika. The experience gained in these isolated skirmishes was all too soon to prove invaluable, for the world was on the brink of greater slaughter than had ever before been envisaged.

CHAPTER 3

Military Hospital Ships, Hospital Carriers and Ambulance Transports from 1914 to 1920

As the title of this chapter indicates, there were different categories of ships in the First World War which were used for roughly similar purposes, and it is as well to begin by mentioning their distinguishing characteristics.

Hospital ships are requisitioned liners, extensively adapted for the particular purpose of aiding the sick and wounded. They are in effect floating hospitals and are medically and surgically equipped to deal with all cases of injury and disease. So that they may be easily distinguished, military hospital ships are painted white overall, with a horizontal band of green, about a metre and a half wide, around the hull. Hospital ships equipped wholly or in part by private individuals or by officially recognized societies are also white but their horizontal band is red. In addition, all have red crosses painted on their sides—fore, aft and amidships—and they fly their national flag as well as the Red Cross flag. To ensure that they are distinguishable at night the hulls are brilliantly illuminated and there are usually long rows or red and green lights along the sides. Identified in this way, they are protected from attack under the Geneva Convention.

Hospital carriers are in effect 'inferior sorts of hospital ships', generally being passenger liners or merchant vessels which have been fitted up as well as time permitted. They carry the distinctive markings of hospital ships and are registered under the Geneva Convention. If from time to time improvements are made ultimately they may become fully fitted-out hospital ships; otherwise they are returned to their former service.

Ambulance transports, while equipped to carry and tend the

sick and wounded, are also used on return journeys to transport troops and stores. The troops, however, can only be accommodated on the decks and are not permitted to use the hospital wards. These vessels do not carry the distinguishing marks of hospital ships and claim no protection under the Geneva Convention. They may be armed to repel attack and use a naval escort when necessary.

As stated, hospital ships enjoy certain protection under the Geneva Convention. This came into being largely as the result of the publication in 1862 of *A Memory in Solferino* written by Jean Henri Dunant, a 34-year-old Swiss industrialist. The First International Conference was held at Geneva the following year and a year later, on 28 August, 1864, a Convention of ten articles applying to land warfare was drawn up.

Then on 20 October, 1868, a Diplomatic Conference was held, again in Geneva, where the first principles were laid down for the adaptation of the first Geneva Convention to maritime warfare. Next came revisions from a conference at the Hague on 29 July, 1899, followed in June, 1906, by another Diplomatic Conference in Geneva whose purpose was to revise the Geneva Convention of 1864. Another Peace Convention was held at the Hague to revise that part of the Convention relating to maritime warfare; this was completed on 17 October, 1907. This adaptation of the Convention laid down the conditions under which hospital ships were entitled to immunity from attack and under which they had to be respected in time of war.

Five military hospital ships were commissioned in the first month of the war. The first three were the *St Andrew,* the *St David* and the *St Patrick,* former cross-channel steamers, each adapted to accommodate about 180 patients. They went to Le Havre on 24 August, their sides painted a dull slate grey; but they were soon given their conventional hospital ship markings. The *St Andrew* made the first voyage carrying 63 lying and 147 sitting casualties who embarked at Rouen. Between that date and 3 September these three vessels, with the much larger hospital ship *Asturias,* made nine journeys from Le Havre or Rouen to Southampton, bringing back a total of 3,387 patients.

The *Asturias* had a chequered career. On 1 August she was

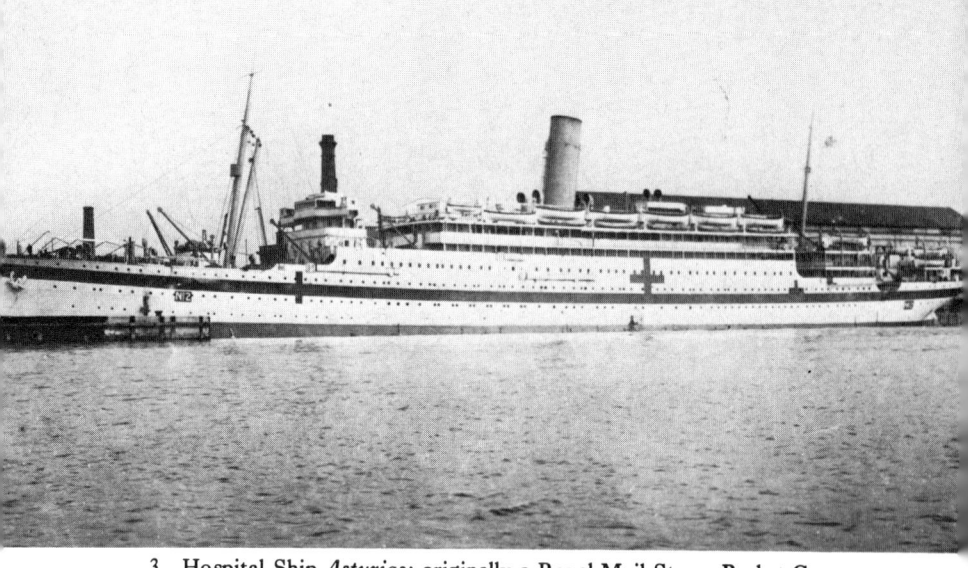

3 Hospital Ship *Asturias*: originally a Royal Mail Steam Packet Company vessel of 12,000 tons, she accommodated 896 patients

mobilized as a naval hospital ship and joined the Grand Fleet at Scapa Flow, but she was soon handed over to the army. On 1 February, 1915, while en route to Le Havre, a German submarine was sighted about 500 yards away and then the track of a torpedo was seen coming directly towards her. The master of the *Asturias* altered course and the weapon missed its mark—all this in broad daylight when the special markings of the hospital ship were clearly visible. She was on regular cross-channel service during the war, and on one occasion when there were extremely heavy casualties at the front she carried 2,400 patients—almost three times her authorized accommodation. In March, 1917, the *Asturias* was again attacked by a U-boat and this time the torpedo struck. She was regarded as a total loss, but was subsequently rebuilt as the cruising liner *Arcadian*.

The *Oxfordshire* was another ship taken over by the navy just before the war, and fitted out as HMHS *No 1*. However, she was found to be too large for naval hospital ship duties and was transferred to the army.

Other military hospital ships which initially served with the navy were the *Guildford Castle*, the *Karapara* and the *Salta*. Many other First World War hospital ships had interesting

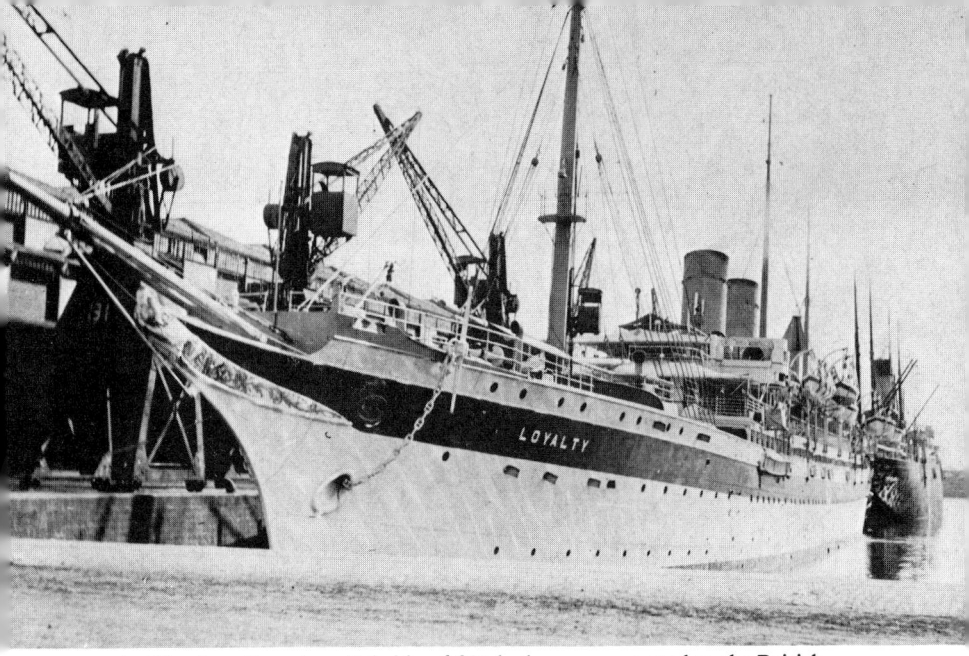

4 The *Loyalty*, a hospital ship of 325 beds, was presented to the British Government in 1914 by the Maharajah of Gwalior and served until 30 November, 1918

backgrounds: the *Glenart Castle* was originally the *Galician* but because the Galicians of the Austro-Hungarian Empire were among Britain's enemies her name was changed. Similarly her sister ship the *German* was renamed the *Glengorm Castle*.

The *Tanda* was made available by the P & O and BI Lines to the people of Madras a few weeks after the outbreak of war when the city decided to provide a hospital ship, and the Company subscribed 20,000 rupees a month towards her upkeep. The *Loyalty* was formerly the *Empress of India* and was sold to the Maharajah of Gwalior for conversion into a hospital ship, while the *Egypt* had served as a hospital ship in the Boer War.

Altogether 77 military hospital ships and transports were commissioned during the war—22 in 1914, 42 in 1915, 7 in 1916 and 6 in 1917. Included in this number were four Belgian Government Mail Steamers—the *Jan Breydel, Pieter de Connick, Stad Antwerpen* and *Ville de Liège*. In addition five yachts were also used for the transport of patients. (Details of these vessels are shown in Appendix E). One other yacht appears to have been employed on hospital ship duties—the Duke of Sutherland's Steam Yacht *Catania*—but she is not officially recorded as doing so.

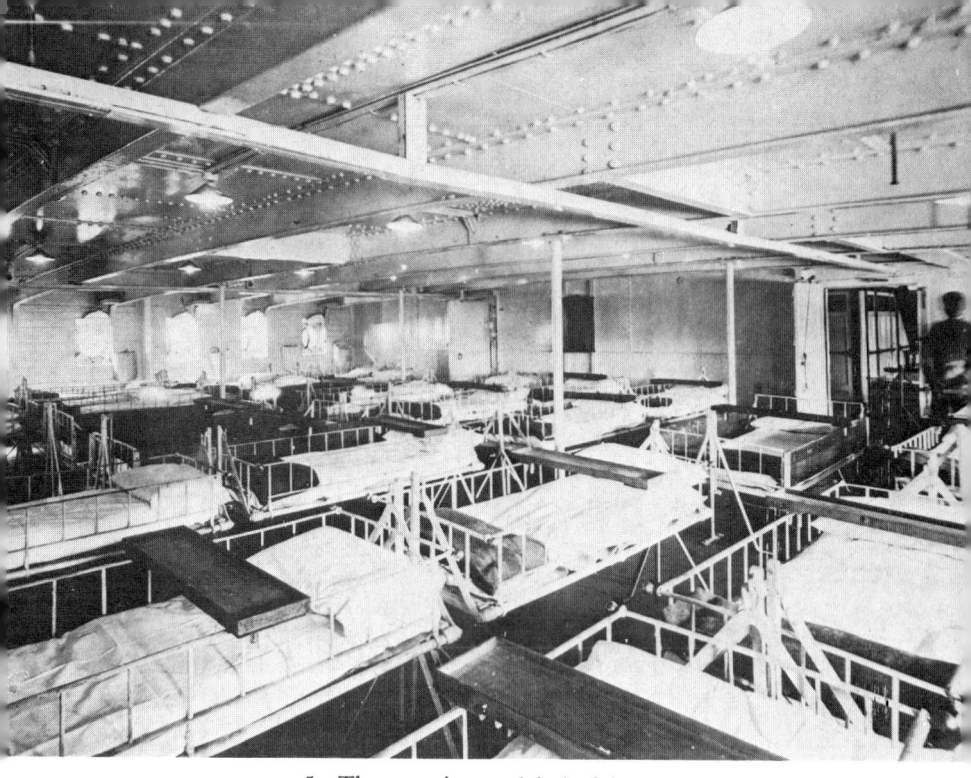

5   The extensive ward deck of the *Loyalty*

6   Hospital Ship *Aquitania,* the first of the three 'great' liners at the Gallipoli campaign, receiving patients from a smaller hospital ship in the Mediterranean

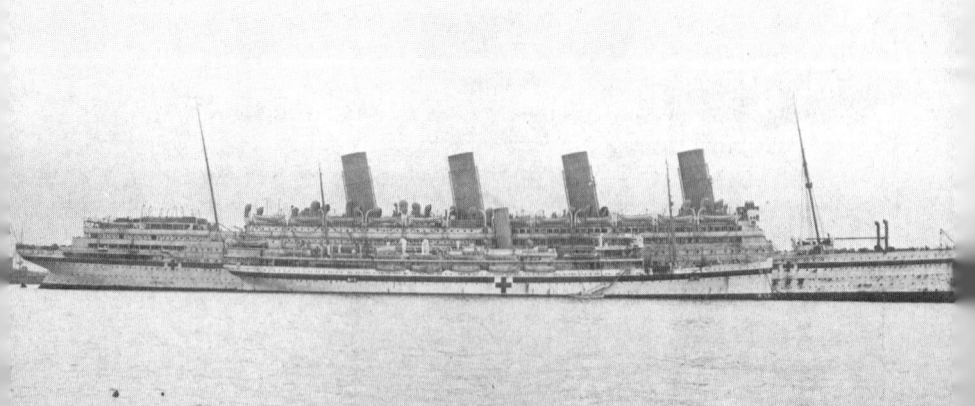

Among the 77 were three of the giant liners of the period. The *Aquitania,* which, with 4,182 beds, had the greatest accommodation of all hospital ships, did just over two years service, from 4 September, 1915, to 27 December, 1917. On one journey from the Dardanelles she had nearly 5,000 patients on board, and 20 ambulance trains were needed to distribute them from Southampton to various hospitals in Britain. The *Britannic* had the second largest accommodation for patients—over 3,300. She was in service for just over a year from 13 November, 1915, her career ending when she struck a mine on 22 November, 1916. The *Mauretania* had room for nearly 2,000 patients but was only employed for four months from 22 November, 1915.

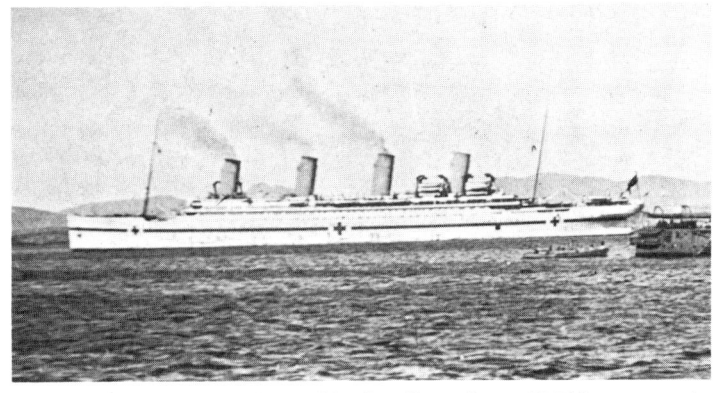

7   Hospital Ship *Britannic,* a White Star liner of over 48,000 tons, was the second 'great' liner at the Gallipoli campaign

At the other end of the scale, a flotilla of six barges—one for personnel, one for stores and four for patients—was formed at Rouen early in the war and designated No. 1 Ambulance Flotilla. The ward barges were each about the size of a Thames lighter and were grouped in pairs—each having 50 beds. But this flotilla was not extensively used. In March, 1915, four additional flotillas were constructed—six barges again being used in each—but the ward barges only had 30 beds. Each of these barges had a kitchen, a dispensary and operating facilities, and was fitted with a generator for electric light. The barges were

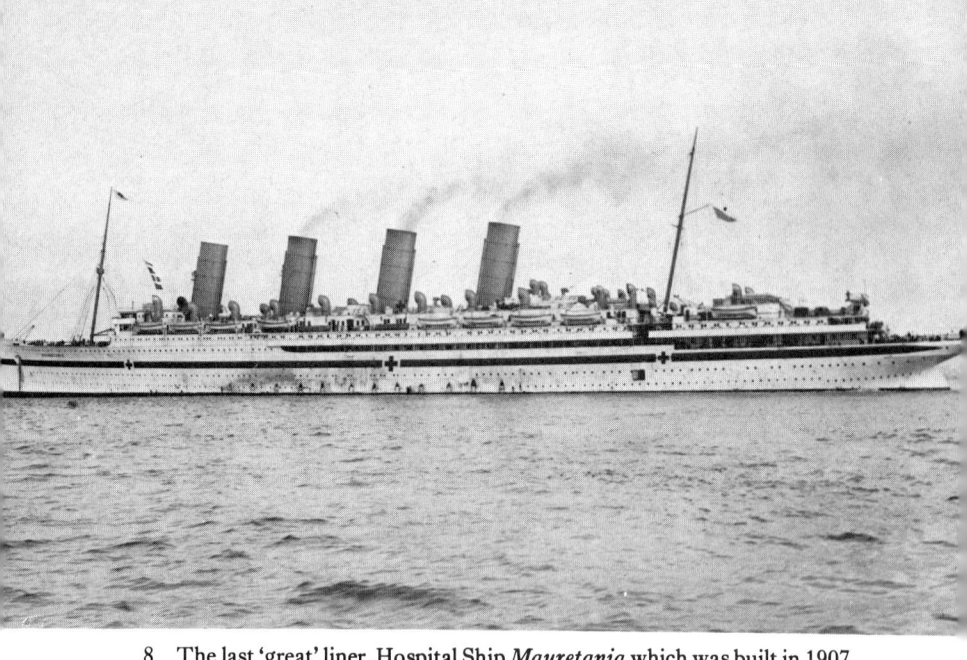

8 The last 'great' liner, Hospital Ship *Mauretania* which was built in 1907 and made three trips from the Dardenelles with patients

intended to carry the more seriously wounded troops, and were towed either singly or in pairs—a medical officer being in charge of each pair of barges.

Patients were carried on stretchers from the canal bank—usually up an unrailed gang plank; from the top of the barge they were lowered by ropes and pulleys to the wards below. The barges moved at about three miles an hour; normally they did not travel at night, and each journey lasted from 24 to 48 hours. They were employed chiefly on the Lys, La Bassée and the Somme canals, and during 1916 these flotillas carried nearly 17,000 patients in 565 barge journeys. In the tragic period of the first battle of the Somme which began on 1 July, 1916, there were 18 barge journeys with 540 patients in the first three days alone. In the whole of the war over 53,000 sick and wounded were transported by barge in France and Flanders.

In the summer of 1915 the British Red Cross Society provided two river motor-launches for Mesopotamia to be used for the evacuation of patients along the Tigris. Previously the casualties had been carried in small clumsy craft—one report saying that they differed little from those in use in about 694

BC! The Society also sent four river motor-launches to the Dardanelles, and at a later date built a fleet of about 60 motor launches—mostly constructed in England, though a few were built in India. Many were sent to Mesopotamia and by the end of 1916 there were 33 BRCS launches in that theatre. A Red Cross river hospital ship, the *Nahba*, reached Basra in May, 1917, having been built in England for service on the Tigris; she made round trips with patients between Basra and Baghdad. Four paddle-steamers were specially built as hospital ships for use by the Inland Water Transport Division in Mesopotamia, and they could each carry 98 British and 96 Indian patients.

Numerous hospital ships were used in the various theatres of

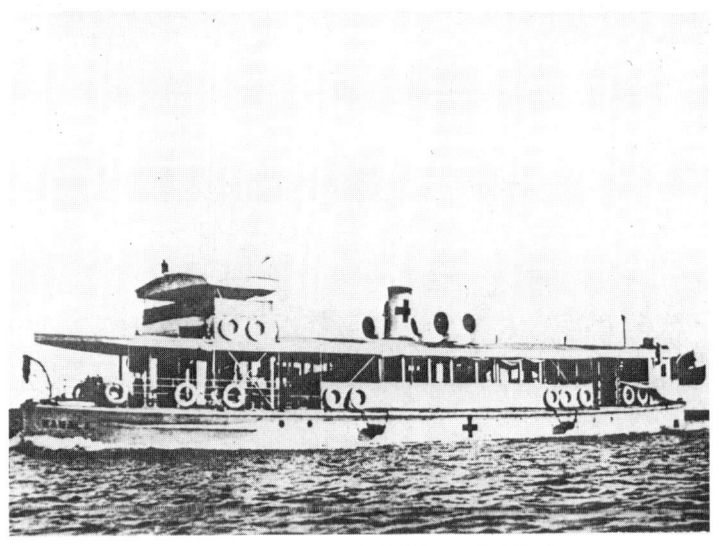

9   River Hospital Ship *Nahba* on the Tigris

the war. The *Franconia* was an ambulance carrier early in 1915 and took 1,614 casualties from Gallipoli to Alexandria. Shortly afterwards, when on other duties, she was torpedoed and sunk in the Mediterranean. In 1916 a small hospital ship called the *Rachid*—formerly an Egyptian customs vessel—carried patients between Mersa Matruh, Alexandria and Sollum.

In the operations against German South-West Africa a hospital transport *City of Athens* and a hospital ship *Ebani* were used, the latter being provided with comforts by the South African Red Cross Society. In an emergency the *Ebani* could carry 500 patients. She was staffed by South African Medical Corps personnel and on the termination of the campaign was handed over to the Imperial authorities.

In the Far East the *Shenking* was fitted out as a hospital ship by the Royal Navy and used for the movement of sick and wounded troops.

The first hospital unit established at the base in the Cameroons was the transport *Assam*—which accommodated 80 European and 300 native patients. She did good service as a base hospital during the first month of the campaign. Of the above six ships, however, only the *Ebani* appears in the official list of military hospital ships.

Among the hospital ships present in the campaign in East Africa were the *Dunluce Castle,* the *Gascon* and the *Guildford Castle.*

Even when the antagonists obeyed the Geneva Convention, hazards still faced the gleaming white hospital ships. In the years 1915–1917 seven military hospital ships struck mines and were either sunk or badly damaged. In 1917 the Central Powers decided to disregard International Law and hospital ships—no matter how prominently marked—were no longer protected by the Geneva Convention. In 1917 and 1918 eight hospital ships were torpedoed. The resulting casualties were indeed tragic.

The *Anglia* was carrying her complement of sick and wounded from Calais to Dover when she struck a mine at about noon on 17 November, 1915. All the patients had life-belts under their pillows and those able to do so put them on, while the staff attended to the others. Splints were removed (if a patient with his legs in wooden splints fell in the water his legs would float and his body would sink) and the walking cases were marshalled on deck, the stretcher patients being carried there. Those patients able to do so threw themselves into the sea; others were lowered down in the life-boats. Of the 388 patients on board 130 were lost, as well as a nursing sister and nine

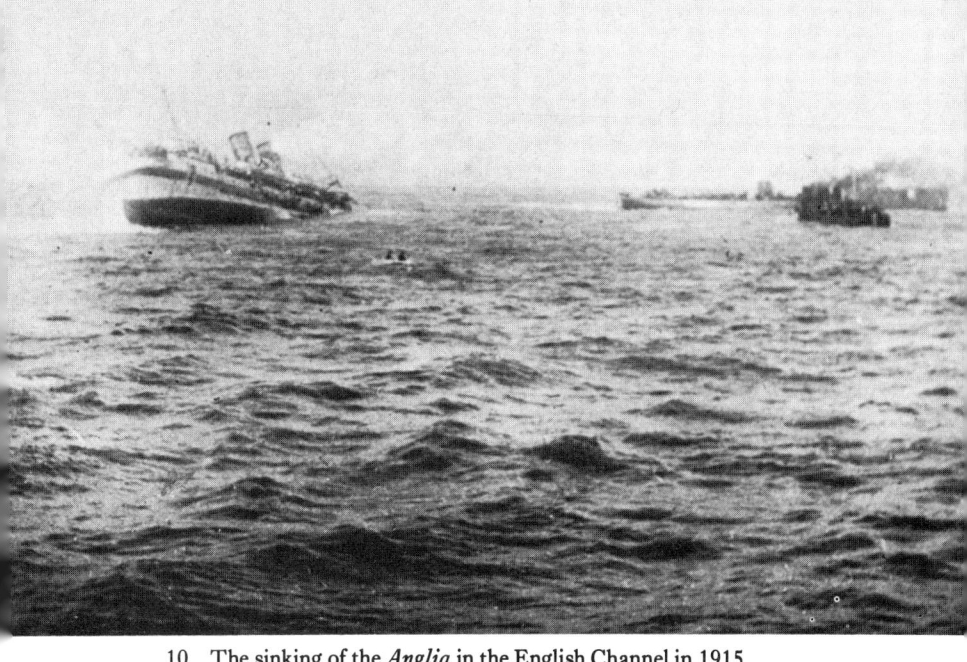

10   The sinking of the *Anglia* in the English Channel in 1915

members of the RAMC. The survivors were picked up by destroyers, patrol boats and other vessels and taken to Dover. A collier, named the *Lusitania,* which went to the rescue unfortunately also struck a mine and sank.

The *Galeka* was mined off Le Havre early in the morning of 28 October, 1916, in a strong gale and heavy sea. Fortunately there were no patients on board, but 19 RAMC personnel were killed by the initial explosion. The remainder of the staff and all the crew were saved, though the vessel was totally wrecked.

The *Britannic* was sunk by a mine at 8.12 am on 21 November, 1916, in the Aegean Sea, on her way to Mudros. The day was warm, there was a calm sea and again no patients were on board. But a medical officer and eight RAMC orderlies were among the 34 fatal casualties out of a total complement of 1,125 crew and medical staff, the latter being made up of 25 medical officers, 76 nursing sisters and 399 RAMC other ranks. The rescue of the survivors was hindered because the great vessel, over 48,000 tons, continued to travel for some distance before sinking.

The *Braemar Castle* also struck a mine in the Aegean Sea, on 23 November, 1916, with the loss of six patients. She was able to continue her duties, however, and her employment in the Russian campaign is mentioned at the end of this chapter.

The *Glenart Castle* was mined both in 1917 and in 1918. She struck a mine at 11.30 pm on 1 March, 1917, en route from Le Havre to Southampton with 520 sick and wounded—300 of whom were cot cases. Fortunately the weather was unusually mild and the sea practically dead calm. All the patients, staff and crew were saved by destroyers, tugs and trawlers; in fact the ship was cleared of invalids by 12.50 am and she was towed into Portsmouth for repairs. Then on 26 February, 1918, she was again mined in the Bristol Channel when on passage to Brest to embark Portuguese sick and wounded. This time she sank in a mere five minutes, and 162 staff and crew lost their lives.

There has already been a brief reference to the ill-fated *Asturias*. She was torpedoed at midnight on 21 March, 1917, when off Start Point on the Devonshire coast, homeward bound from Salonika. There were no patients on board, but a medical officer, a nursing sister and 12 RAMC orderlies were drowned, as well as 29 of the ship's company (including a stewardess). She was beached at Salcombe and eventually towed to Plymouth. When attacked, the *Asturias* had all her lights on and the red crosses illuminated. Soon after this sinking the conventional hospital ship markings were abandoned in home waters and the vessels 'dazzle-painted'. They subsequently sailed as ambulance transports and were provided with a gun for defence.

The *Gloucester Castle,* which, in the earlier days of the war, had served in the Gallipoli campaign, was torpedoed in the English channel at 7 pm on 30 March, 1917. She was carrying 399 sick and wounded from Le Havre to Southampton—300 being cot cases. All but one were saved by destroyers and transports, but three died during the transfer. The vessel was eventually brought into port about a fortnight later.

On the morning of 10 April, 1917, the *Salta* was mined just outside Le Havre but she had no patients on board. The Commanding Officer, four medical officers, nine nursing sisters, 37 RAMC orderlies and two of the crew were lost with the ship, which sank rapidly.

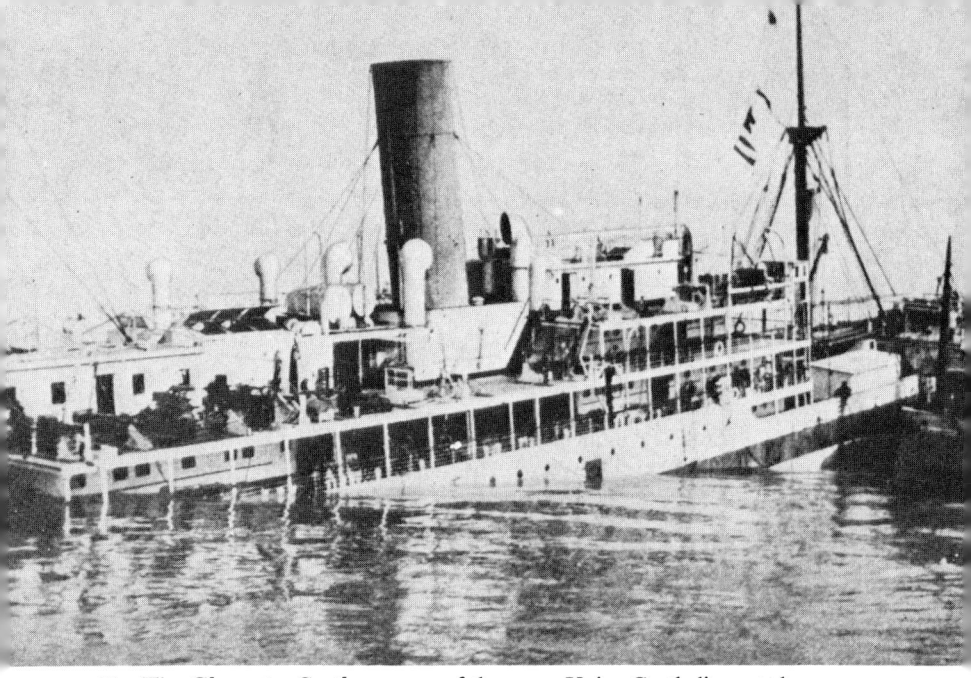

11 The *Gloucester Castle* was one of the many Union Castle liners to be converted into a hospital ship during the First World War. She is seen here after being torpedoed

17 April, 1917, was a fateful day for ambulance transports—both the *Lanfranc* and the *Donegal* being torpedoed by the enemy and sunk on that day. The *Lanfranc*, while carrying 387 patients, 167 of whom were Germans, was attacked north of Le Havre at 7.30 pm. There were 326 cot cases among the patients, many of whom were seriously wounded, including a number of amputations and fractured femurs. Seventeen British and the same number of German patients were lost and the ship sank rapidly. A similar fate befell the *Donegal* which was distinctively marked when she was attacked but her whereabouts at the time is not officially recorded. Fortunately she was carrying only slightly wounded patients, 29 of whom, together with 12 of her crew, were reported 'missing'.

Another hospital ship which was torpedoed without warning was the *Dover Castle*—at 11 am on 26 May, 1917, in the Mediterranean. All the 632 patients on board were saved; so, apparently, were all the staff and crew, though three of the ship's life-boats were destroyed by the first explosion. The hospital ship *Karapara* took 270 survivors to Gibraltar, and after the stricken ship had been completely cleared, she was sunk by a second torpedo.

The *Goorkha* was mined at 11.50 am on 10 October, 1917, off Malta. There were 362 patients on board, including 17 nursing sisters. The vessel was cleared in 35 minutes and there were no casualties; she was subsequently towed into Malta harbour.

The *Guildford Castle* had a lucky escape when she was struck by a torpedo on 10 March, 1918. The torpedo did not explode and the vessel made port safely.

The circumstances of the torpedoing of the *Llandovery Castle* are tragic. She was only completed in 1914 and, when in use as a hospital ship by the Canadian forces in June, 1918, was sailing from Halifax to Liverpool. She was carrying no patients but her complement of 258 included many Canadian nursing sisters. At 9.30 on the night of 27 June, 1918, when 118 miles west of Fastnet, she was torpedoed and sunk without warning by a German submarine. A number of lifeboats and rafts were launched but the U boat—by shelling and by ramming—sank all but one. In the darkness, only one boat, with the 24 sole survivors, escaped. Eighty-eight medical staff and 146 crew were lost in one of the most savage acts at sea throughout the First World War.

The hospital ship *Warilda* was torpedoed in the English Channel at 1.30 am on 3 August, 1918, when returning from Le Havre. Of the 471 sick and wounded on board, 439 were cot cases. The losses were very heavy—115 patients, one nursing sister and an RAMC orderly. The rest of the patients, staff and crew were cleared from the ship within an hour. She sank 30 minutes later.

The first torpedoing of a British hospital ship—the *Asturias*—occurred on 21 March, 1917. There is, however, a record that a Russian hospital ship, the *Portugal,* was torpedoed off the Turkish coast a year earlier, on 17 March, 1916. This vessel, which fortunately had no patients on board, was flying a Red Cross flag and had red crosses painted on her funnels. She was destroyed with the loss of 85 lives. Of these 25 were nurses and 24 others were members of the Red Cross staff. Another Russian hospital ship, the *Vpered,* was sunk on 10 July, 1916, while the *Koningin Regentes,* a Dutch hospital ship, was sunk either by mine or torpedo on 31 January, 1917.

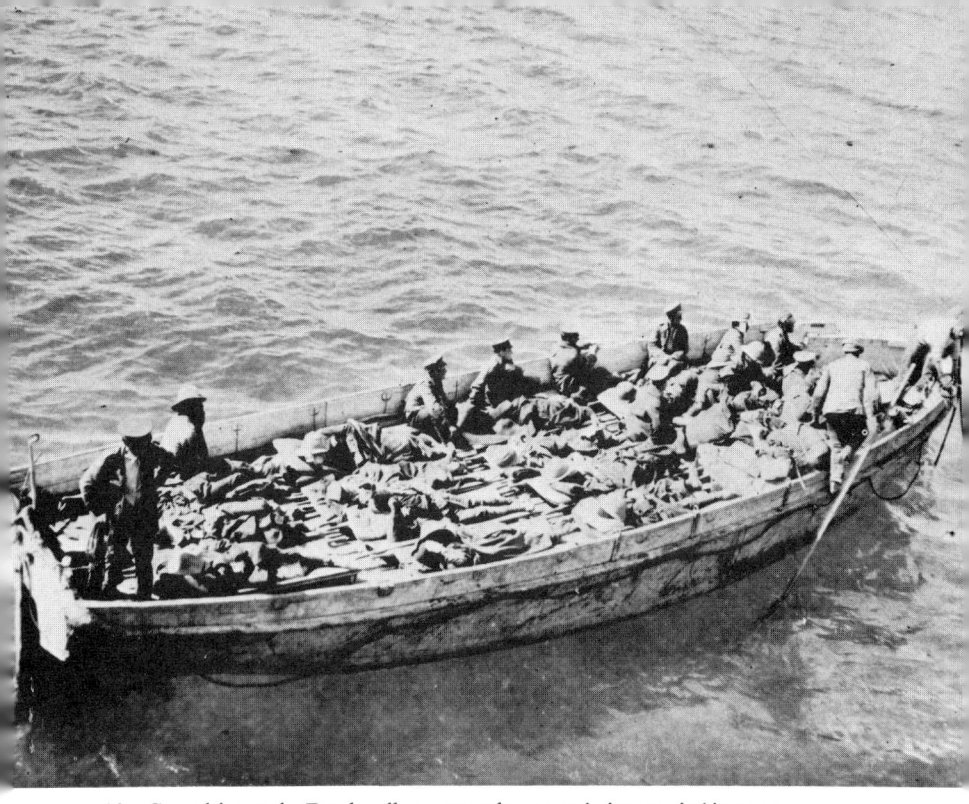

12 Casualties at the Dardenelles—stretcher cases being carried in an open boat to the military hospital ship *Dongola* in 1915

Special reference must be made to the very important part which hospital ships, troopships and transports played in the treatment and movement of the sick and wounded during the Gallipoli campaign, from the first landings on 25 April, 1915, to the final evacuation which ended on 10 January, 1916. At least 22 hospital ships and some 20 troopships, transports and similar vessels took part at some period and took casualties to Imbros, Mudros, Alexandria, Malta and elsewhere. The names of these vessels are given in Appendix D.

For considerable periods during the campaign these vessels lay off-shore and casualties were towed to them in smaller craft from the beaches. In the early days this was by naval tow of small boats each carrying about 30 patients. Later on, as soon as a troopship landed its complement on the beaches, or transports unloaded their cargoes, the empty vessels were at once filled with casualties. The patients were cleared with the least possible delay because their great numbers practically stopped all operational work on the beaches. These 'carriers' then moved to the hospital or other ships lying off-shore and transferred the casualties.

At a later stage mine-sweepers were brought into use for evacuating casualties. They were partly fitted for medical purposes and each carried medical officers and orderlies. Of the eight railway steam packets commissioned by the Admiralty and officially called 'fleet mine-sweepers' five were used for these duties; they were the *Clacton, Hythe, Newmarket, Redbreast* and one other whose name has not been recorded.

The British Red Cross Society also provided six specially equipped 'pulling' motor launches for the evacuation from the Gallipoli beaches, and each had accommodation for 12 serious or 36 light cases.

A number of merchant vessels were set aside for the reception of the sick and wounded, and they were often called hospital ships even before they had been painted white. Because of the colour of their hulls they were later called 'black ships' and were easily identified from the 'white' hospital ships which had the conventional colours. The terms 'white' and 'black' ships were subsequently taken into general use in this theatre of war.

The magnitude of the task undertaken by these vessels during the Gallipoli campaign was tremendous: during the nine months April to December, 1915, nearly 110,000 sick and wounded were evacuated to Egypt; in August, September and October of the same year over 50,000 patients were carried to Malta, Gibraltar and the United Kingdom; in a ten-day period during the evacuation from 11 to 20 December, 1915, nearly 84,000 patients were re-embarked from Suvla and Anzac and taken to Imbros and Mudros.

The medical history of the Gallipoli campaign also reflects quite clearly the invaluable and very considerable part played by the Army Medical Services of Australia and of New Zealand.

After the defeat of the Central Powers came the intervention in Northern Russia, and early in 1918 the *Braemar Castle* went to Murmansk, where she was used as a base hospital. To provide increased accommodation, and also to keep out the cold, her decks were boarded-in and she became known as the

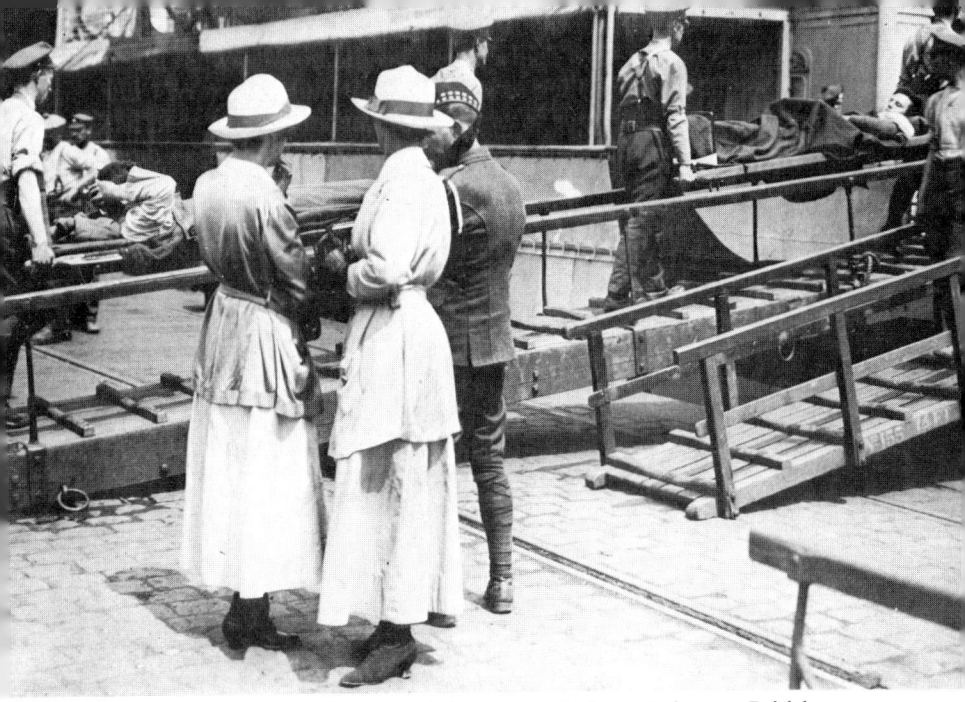

13 Stretcher cases being carried from an ambulance train to a British hospital ship at Boulogne in May, 1918

'Noah's Ark'. She was in Murmansk for nearly a year, packed in by ice which was broken up by Russian refugees as it threatened to 'pinch' the ship. When the campaign there ended the *Braemar Castle* was sent to Leith in a convoy. She then went to Archangel and was the last vessel to leave that port when it was evacuated.

The *Kalyan,* having been used for troop carrying between England, Egypt and Salonika, was converted into a hospital ship and sailed for North Russia in October, 1918. She reached Archangel after a 12-day voyage and on arrival made fast to a berth in the Dvina estuary—remaining there for eight months. She acted as a temporary base hospital for British, American, French, Italian, Chinese and Russian sick and wounded, who reached her by barge from the mainland. When winter came the Dvina froze solid, and within a week a railway line had been laid on the frozen surface; the casualties then arrived by ambulance trains. Many patients were also taken to the *Kalyan* by sleighs, but in April, 1919, the ice began to melt and the ship returned to Leith early in June.

In May, 1919, two paddle-steamers, the *Walton Belle* and the *London Belle* were fitted out as hospital tenders and spent four months at Archangel ferrying wounded from the Russian campaign to homeward-bound hospital ships.

The amount of work done by hospital ships and similar vessels in the First World War was vast: the total number of sick and wounded who arrived in Britain from all fronts from August, 1914 to August, 1920, was 2,655,025; and during the same period it took 776 hospital-ship journeys to carry more than 194,000 patients from Mediterranean garrisons and theatres of war to the British Isles.

CHAPTER 4

Naval and Military Hospital Ships and Carriers in the Second World War

The many developments in medicine and in shipbuilding and engineering led to a greater use of carriers in the Second World War than in the First. The totally different type of warfare fought from 1939 to 1945 called for a much closer cooperation between the forces, and naval and military hospital ships were frequently used together, quite a number also being transferred from one service to another.

During the brief Norway campaign from April to June, 1940, the hospital ships *Aba* and *Atlantis* evacuated casualties. This also appears to be the first occasion in which hospital ships carried officers of the Army Dental Corps.

In the miraculous evacuation of Dunkirk a number of railway-owned steamers were converted into hospital carriers, but before the final beach-head was reached, one of these, the *Brighton*, ran regularly between Dieppe and Newhaven —sometimes with over 250 patients on board. She never saw the final stages of the evacuation, however, for she was sunk in an air raid on 21 May, 1940—the same day as the *Maid of Kent* was bombed and sunk at Dieppe, even though she bore the unmistakable markings of a hospital carrier.

The *Paris* was the only hospital carrier to enter Calais during the May retreat and she evacuated 349 casualties. Altogether she made five entries into Calais where her crew went ashore to search for wounded and then acted as stretcher bearers to get them on board. She was also active at Dunkirk, where she embarked 740 patients on 29 May, 1940. When making her sixth outward voyage on 2 June, 1940, she was bombed and sank off Dunkirk.

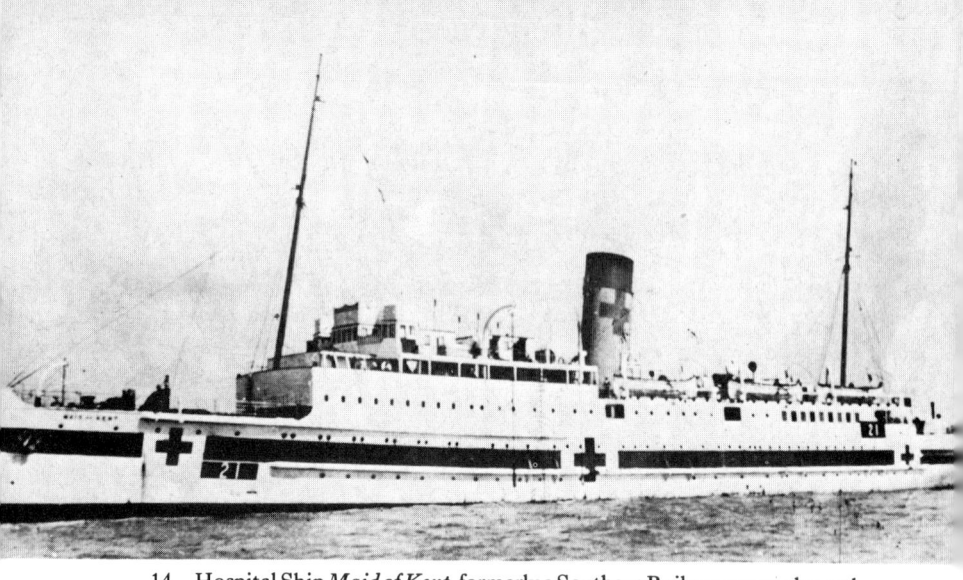

14 Hospital Ship *Maid of Kent*, formerly a Southern Railway cross-channel steamer, which was bombed and sunk off Dieppe in May, 1940

The *Isle of Jersey* and the *Dinard* both became hospital carriers early in the war and the record of the latter was exceptionally good; after rescuing 371 men from Dunkirk she was for a time used as a floating hospital for merchant seamen whose vessels had been sunk by enemy aircraft.

The *St Julien* made a number of trips with casualties from Dieppe and Boulogne and she was in the thick of the fray at Dunkirk, being repeatedly attacked from the air and by shore batteries. She made six attempts to enter the port and twice succeeded in rescuing wounded. Later she carried casualties from Cherbourg to Newhaven and was then transferred to Scotland.

The *St Andrew* and the *St David* also shared the perils of Dunkirk where their crews volunteered to help rescue the wounded. The *St Helier* and the *Roebuck* both merit mention for their work in the evacuation of casualties; the former lay in Dunkirk harbour on 1 June, 1940, and loaded 40 stretcher cases, while the *Roebuck* embarked 47 stretcher cases, 72 other wounded and some fit troops, all of whom were landed at Dover on 1 June.

Ten hospital carriers which were converted railway steamers were based at Newhaven, the No 1 Ambulance Port

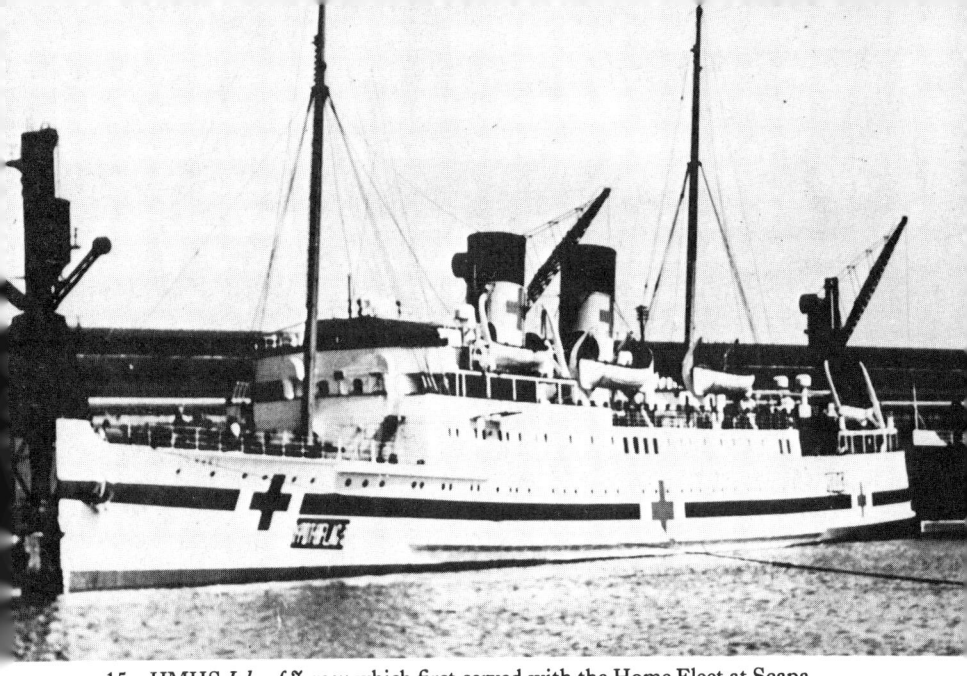

15 HMHS *Isle of Jersey* which first served with the Home Fleet at Scapa Flow and subsequently operated as one of a pool of military hospital carriers on the Anzio and Normandy beaches. She was originally a Southern Railways vessel

16 Hospital Ship *St Julien* was originally a Great Western Railway steamer which was converted into a military hospital ship of 220 beds. She was in the thick of the fray at Dunkirk where she was at one time under fire from both the air and from shore batteries

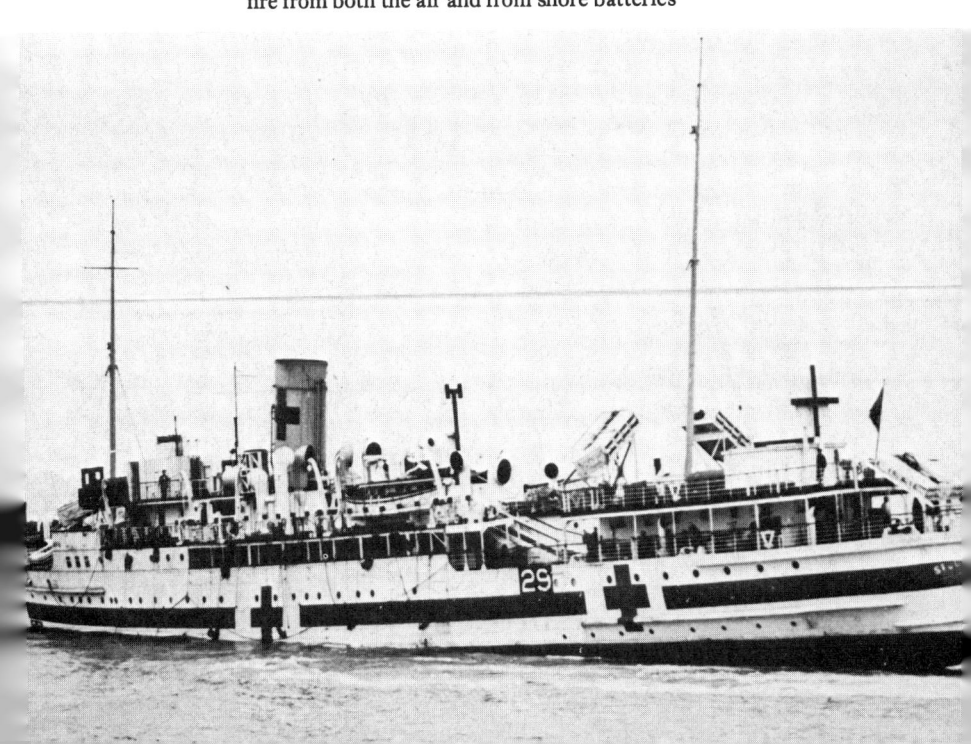

for the British Expeditionary Force. During the Dunkirk evacuation this small fleet brought more than 20,000 casualties to the United Kingdom.

In November, 1940, the hospital carrier *Leinster* went to Iceland, first to Reykjavik and then to Akureyri, where she spent the whole of the winter. In the neighbourhood of Narvik a Norwegian ship was converted into a hospital carrier and on one occasion embarked casualties from two British battleships south of the port.

A year later, on 6 December, 1941, the hospital ship *Somersetshire* reached Tobruk and anchored about $1\frac{1}{4}$ miles from the shore. The patients were brought to the ship by two motor launches each towing three life-boats which had accommodation for nine stretcher and two or three sitting cases. It took two days to embark 540 patients and, during the night, the *Somersetshire* was under bombardment for over eleven hours. She later took part in the invasion of Sicily, embarked 600 sick and wounded at Syracuse and took them to Alexandria.

The *Atlantis,* two years after Norway, attended the Madagascar campaign in May, 1942, transporting casualties from the island to Durban. (In 1945 she took a full load of sick and wounded American troops from Europe to New York.)

The *Llandovery Castle* went to Tobruk after the victory at El Alamein; she arrived in November, 1942, and embarked 715 casualties for Alexandria.

A number of the carriers which had been at Dunkirk served in the Mediterranean in 1943–1944, where they assisted the amphibious operations by following the main landing forces and getting as close inshore as possible. To enable casualties to be taken off the beaches they were equipped with 'water-ambulances' which took the place of lifeboats. These were specially fitted to take stretcher cases and were slung out and down into the sea by electrically operated davits; when they returned with patients they were winched up and the unloading carried out on deck. The water-ambulances had powerful engines and were constructed of light wood; and, being flat-bottomed, they could run right on to the beach.

In April, 1943, an exchange of seriously ill and wounded British and Italian prisoners-of-war was arranged under the

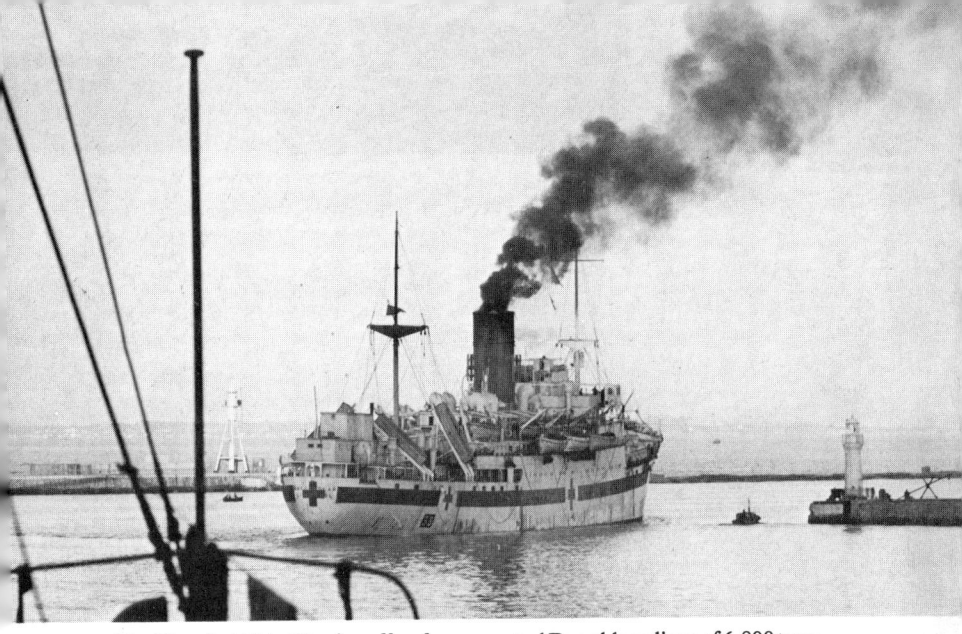

17 Hospital Ship *Newfoundland*, a converted Donaldson liner of 6,800 tons leaving Salerno harbour. She was attacked and sunk off the Salerno beaches in 1943

provisions of Article 68 of the Geneva Convention; the British contingent went to Lisbon by rail where they were exchanged for Italians, who had arrived in the hospital ship *Newfoundland*—in which the British were then taken back to the United Kingdom.

Mention of the *Newfoundland* introduces a further mention of the *Leinster*—a lively and detailed account written by Geraldine Edge and Mary Johnston, two of the nursing sisters on the ship, in their book *The Ships of Youth*. As Hospital Carrier No 37, the *Leinster* left Scotland for the Mediterranean on 25 June, 1943, with four other carriers. The book records the sinking of the *Newfoundland* which, in company with the *Leinster* and *St Andrew* and *Tairea*, was ordered to leave the vicinity of the Salerno beaches where there was continuous air bombardment. They were to proceed to sea and, when outside the five mile limit, were to be fully illuminated as hospital ships and carriers, and so obtain protection under the Geneva Convention. But in the middle of the night of 13 September, 1943, when about 25 miles off Salerno, they were attacked by enemy aircraft and the *Newfoundland* received a direct hit which smashed all but one of the lifeboats; it also put the pumps out of order and the fire which started could not be controlled. Five medical officers, six nursing sisters, eight RAMC

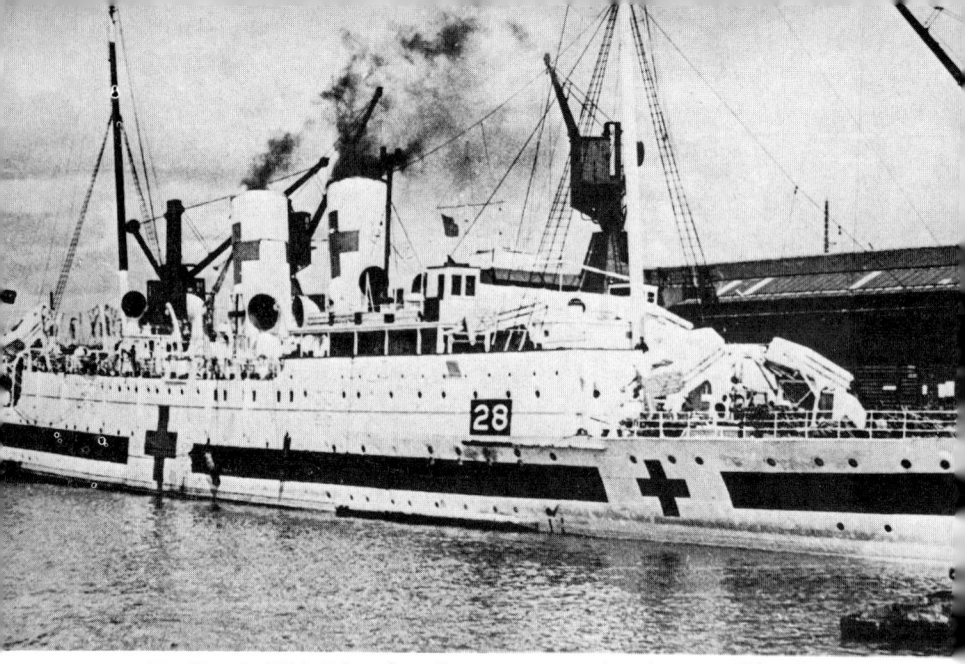

18 Hospital Ship *Dinard*, a railway steamer equipped to carry 220 patients. She collected casualties from the Normandy and Anzio beaches and remained in service despite being mined

orderlies and 19 of the crew lost their lives. The *St Andrew* picked up about 100 survivors who were mostly American nurses, while the *Leinster* rescued 60, many of whom were badly wounded. The *Leinster* herself was in trouble some time later, in Anzio Bay, when on 25 January, 1944, she was repeatedly hit by bombs. Although set on fire she managed to survive. During the time she was in the area she made 35 journeys from Anzio, carrying out 20,800 casualties.

Both the hospital carriers *Dinard* and *St Julien* did good work in the Italian campaign area during 1943–1944, the former visiting 30 ports, steaming over 30,000 miles and carrying nearly 7,600 patients. The *St Julien,* which covered a similar distance, also helped to recover casualties from the Anzio beaches.

The *St Andrew* and the *St David* are two other vessels which deserve special mention. They reached the Mediterranean in June, 1943, in time for the landings at Salerno, and made many journeys between Italian ports and Malta and North Africa, sometimes steaming over 1,000 miles on one trip. They were both frequently attacked from the air and eventually the *St David* was sunk 25 miles south of Anzio on 25 January, 1944, with the loss of 55 lives. Among the dead were the skipper, the commanding officer and another medical officer, and two nursing sisters. During her period in the Mediterranean the *St David* had carried 6,000 patients and had travelled some 25,000 miles. The *St Andrew* picked up many of the survivors from her sister ship and eventually made 37 trips to Anzio, later carrying casualties from Ancona to Bari. In September, 1944, on her last scheduled voyage between these ports, she struck a mine but was towed into Taranto for repairs; she was subsequently brought back to Birkenhead for a complete overhaul.

The military hospital ship *Talamba,* which was also engaged in these operations, was bombed and sunk off Sicily. Other hospital ships present included the naval hospital ships *Aba, Amarapoora, Oxfordshire* and *Vita* while the United States provided the *Acadia, Seminole* and *Shamrock.* In addition a 'personnel' ship, the *Arcadian,* was specially 'staffed and stored' as a casualty station ship for Oran.

Railway-owned steamers continued their work as hospital carriers in the Normandy landings. The *Amsterdam* made two trips to France, but in August, 1944, was sunk by a mine off the French coast with a tragically heavy loss of patients, staff and crew. The *Dinard* began to collect early casualties from the beaches on 7 July, 1944, but struck a mine and was towed back to Southampton for repairs. She subsequently returned to hospital carrier service, and by December she had made 37 trips across the channel and had carried 6,700 patients. The *Isle of Jersey,* formerly a naval hospital ship with the Home Fleet, was included in a pool of miliary hospital carriers operating the Normandy beaches; between 8 June and 16 July this pool of carriers evacuated 20,000 casualties.

Two exchanges of sick and wounded prisoners took place in 1944, one at Barcelona where 900 patients were embarked on the *Gripsholm,* and the other at Göthenberg when three vessels were needed to carry home 3,000 prisoners-of-war and 600 interned civilians.

The use of Royal Naval Hospital Ships in the Second World War is covered in great detail in the *Medical History of the Second World War—Royal Naval Medical Services,* which is the source of much of the information in the remainder of this chapter. But it is worthwhile to once more emphasize the essential differences between military and naval hospital ships. As in the First World War, the military vessel was essentially a link in the lines of medical communication and chiefly carried patients from one port to another. But the naval hospital ship was not only required to be the equivalent of a field hospital but also be capable of serving as a base hospital. It had to be able to keep within reasonable distance of the Fleet or its replenishing group, and at times had to expand its sick accommodation by converting its single berths into doubles when carrying patients to a base or to the United Kingdom.

HMHS *Maine* was already in service with the navy before the war broke out and in August, 1939, she was augmented by the *Isle of Jersey*, which, after service at Dunkirk, was mainly used as a base hospital at Scapa Flow before being attached to the fleet of military carriers for the Normandy invasion in June, 1944.

Next to be taken into service was the *Aba* which was converted for hospital ship duties in September, 1939. Six months later she was transferred to the army and went to Norway.

The *Amarapoora*, requisitioned in September, 1939, was also used on base hospital duties and in April, 1940, embarked casualties from the Norway campaign. She was then used on carrier duties between North Africa and the United Kingdom. On 13 September, 1943, when anchored off Salerno with other hospital ships, she was attacked by enemy aircraft; this was the occasion when the military hospital ship *Newfoundland* was sunk. Afterwards she went to Glasgow, where on 12 November she had a refit and her accommodation increased by 100 beds. This was followed by another spell in the Mediterranean, by further base hospital duty at Scapa Flow, and then by service in the Far East. (On 13 August, 1946, she was paid off by the Navy and handed over to the Army.)

Next to join the Royal Navy was the *Vasna*, which was commissioned at Bombay in September, 1939, and attached to the East Indies Squadron. She was in the Mediterranean early in 1940 and was also at the evacuation of Norway; she was hit in the Liverpool blitz in December that year. The *Vasna* joined the South Atlantic Squadron in Freetown in 1941, and returned

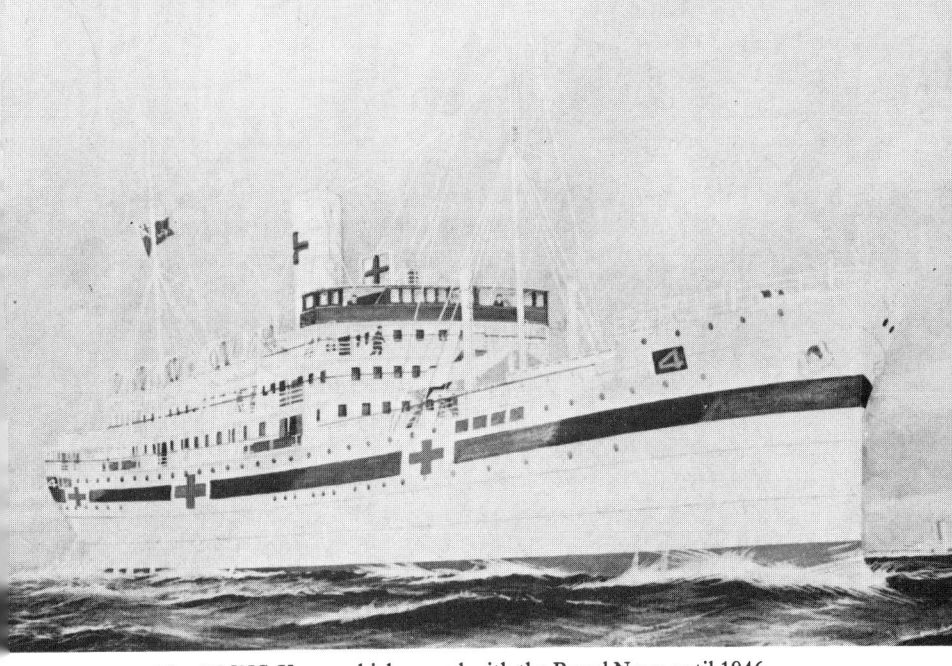

19 HMHS *Vasna* which served with the Royal Navy until 1946

to the Home Fleet in July. She then joined the Eastern Fleet at Ceylon in February, 1942, and in October covered the landings on Madagascar. In June, 1943, she was seconded for service with the army for operations in the Mediterranean, being based at Tripoli for the Sicily landings and then going to the Persian Gulf before rejoining the Eastern Fleet at Trincomalee. In September, 1944, the *Vasna* went to work on the Burma coast, and by 21 January, 1945, she was at Akyab, covering the landings on Ramree Island and on Cheduba Island five days later. After a visit to South Africa she once more joined the Eastern Fleet in June and ended the war with the British Pacific Fleet. After the war she was employed in the recuperation of prisoners-of-war from Japanese camps and, as the only British hospital ship in Japanese waters, she acted as the Fleet hospital. She went to Okinawa in October and took ex-prisoners-of-war to Sydney.

The *Oxfordshire* was employed as a base hospital at Freetown from November, 1939, to February, 1941, this period including a refit at Port Elizabeth. After a brief spell in home waters she went to North Africa for the Allied invasion and remained there until June, 1943; for the rest of that year she did carrier duties in the area. The *Oxfordshire* had a second refit early in 1944, at Swansea, and was involved in the Anzio operations. She then went to Clydebank in Scotland where she was fitted with a new ward of 86 beds before being sent to Scapa Flow. This was followed by duty with the Pacific Fleet Train, and by secondment to the United States Seventh Fleet as base hospital ship at Subic Bay before she returned to Liverpool for release on 5 December, 1945.

The *Vita* was requisitioned in May, 1940, and was converted at Bombay on 3 August. Her first trip with patients was from Berbera to Aden and Bombay, and from September until February, 1941, she was base hospital ship at Aden. Later, when loaded with over 400 casualties, she was attacked by nine enemy aircraft while lying off Tobruk. Fortunately she did not receive a direct hit, but a near miss lifted her stern completely out of the water and this damaged the superstructure, put both engines and dynamos out of action, wrecked five wards and set the laboratory and dispensary on fire. A serious list to port developed and the patients and most of the medical and nursing staff were evacuated to HMAS *Waterhen;* the Principal Medical Officer and remaining medical staff and the ship's officers were taken off when the vessel seemed about to founder. But a few hours later, although still under enemy aircraft attack, the *Vita* was still afloat and it was possible to tow her into harbour. She remained under frequent attack, but on 21 April was towed to Port Said, being bombed twice on the voyage. Eventually she got through the Suez canal to Port Tewfik where she had minor repairs and was rejoined by her staff and crew. The long-suffering *Vita* then made passage to Bombay, running on only one engine and without light or ventilation since the dynamos were still out of action. When repairs and refitting were completed she returned to Aden, but was at Addu Atoll in November, 1941, and at Colombo on New Year's Day, 1942. The *Vita* then returned to Addu Atoll where on 8 April, 1943, she was in the vicinity of two British warships sunk by enemy aircraft. Honouring her status, the Japanese stopped their attacks when she reached the scene of the disaster and she was able to embark 595 survivors, who were landed at Colombo on 10 April. Six days later she was once more at Addu

Atoll and again embarked casualties from sunken British warships, this time taking them to Durban, which was reached on 31 May. Base hospital duties at Kilindini followed after which she had a refit at Bombay, leaving there on 27 September for carrier duties at Diego Suarez. The *Vita* underwent a refit at Bombay and did duty with the Eastern Fleet in January, 1944, before returning again to the dockyard at Bombay. Base hospital duties at Trincomalee were followed by acting as a carrier between Colombo and Durban, but by April, 1945, she was at Cochin, Southern India. On 28 April she called at Kyankpyu and in May took army casualties from Rangoon to Calcutta. The pursuit of the Japanese from Burma was at that time at its height, and the *Vita* made a journey to Chittagong where she embarked casualties for Madras. This was followed by a further spell as base hospital at Trincomalee, before she made her last visit to Bombay for yet another refit. Her busy career as a hospital ship ended in January, 1946, when she was paid off.

Two Dutch vessels, the three year old *Tjitjalengka* and the seventeen year old *Ophir*, were requisitioned from the Netherlands Ministry of Shipping and Fisheries on 8 July, 1942, and the newer ship was converted at Liverpool. In October she carried American and Canadian invalids to Halifax, Nova Scotia, and then worked as a base hospital at Freetown until February, 1943. After service in the Indian Ocean the *Tjitjalengka* moved to Trincomalee in December, 1943, for base duty, after which she sailed to Sydney to serve with the Eastern Fleet in the Pacific. In June, 1945, she was loaned to the United States as a temporary base hospital ship at Leyte. She returned to the Eastern Fleet Train in mid-July and after the war went to Yokohama to embark ex-prisoners of war for New Zealand. At Shanghai she embarked ex-internees and then went to Singapore to pick up a group of invalids and took all her patients to Madras. She then sailed for the United Kingdom, on the way embarking patients at Colombo and Durban for disembarkation at Tilbury, London, before going to Liverpool, where she was released.

The conversion of the *Ophir* started at Calcutta and was completed at Colombo. She began her hospital ship duties at

Addu Atoll on 27 January, 1943, and returned to Colombo in May. She then did a carrier trip to Suez, and on 19 June joined the Mediterranean Fleet, but was back in the Indian Ocean with the Eastern Fleet at Bombay in August, doing carrier duties with army invalids. A period was spent on repairs at Bombay, and the *Ophir* remained in that area doing carrier work until 1 June, 1945, when she went to the Mediterranean to bring Indian army patients from Taranto to Bombay. Base hospital duties at Trincomalee were followed by similar employment at Port Swettenham during the re-occupation of Malaya. After the war, on 14 October, she sailed via Singapore for Batavia, and during this voyage the Dutch officers and crew made a successful search for their families who had been held by the Japanese. After carrying invalids from Port Swettenham and Madras to Calcutta she was paid off at that port in April, 1946.

A French vessel, the *Cap St Jacques,* had been converted into an army hospital ship in 1944 and was transferred to the navy in April, 1945. Her initial voyage was to carry 400 patients for repatriation, 75 being disembarked at Suez and the rest at Ceylon in June. She went to Durban for alterations and repairs in October and although she only made short carrier trips in the following months, some repairs were necessary at each port. In 1946 she assisted in the repatriation of Allied prisoners of war from Singapore and took French invalids from Saigon to Toulon. She was handed back to her owners on 18 April, 1946.

An Italian passenger liner, the *Gerusalemme,* was requisitioned by the Admiralty in January, 1945, and converted at Durban. She started hospital ship duties at the end of July when she reached Manus, Admiralty Island, but a fire on board soon put her out of action. In the following September she did local duty during the relief of Hong Kong and finished as a temporary base hospital ship at Singapore early in 1946.

This chapter has already shown that many military hospital ships used Indian ports during the war, and the *Karapara, Karoa, Tairea, Talamba* and *Wu Sueh* also did so. A number of hospital river steamers were also used in India—these vessels being adapted to carry up to 100 patients.

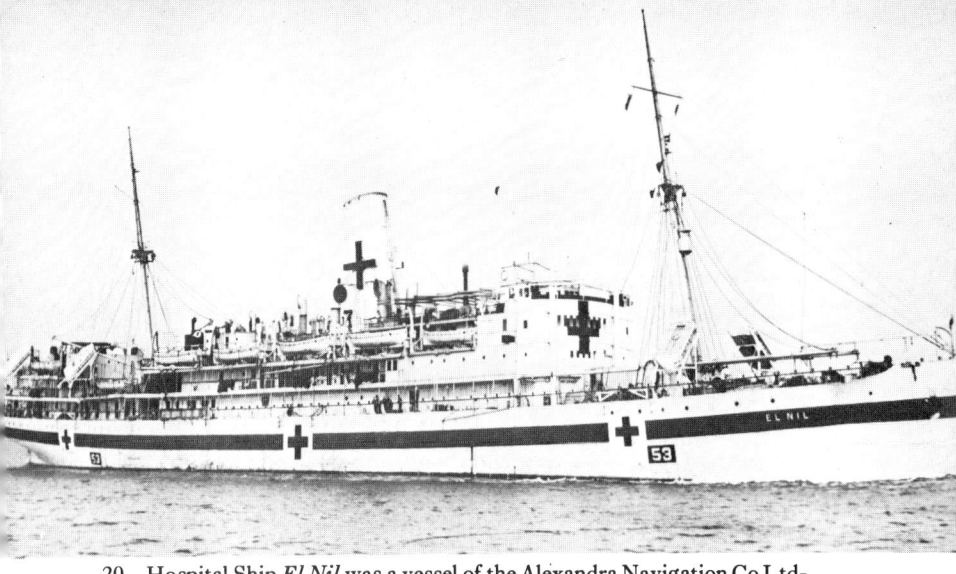

20 Hospital Ship *El Nil* was a vessel of the Alexandra Navigation Co Ltd-Furness Withy (M) Line that was employed on special time duty from May, 1944 until late 1947. She carried some 28,000 patients during her fifty-two recorded voyages

Details of sixty of the military and naval hospital ships and carriers in service during the Second World War are shown in Appendix E, while a table which gives the numbers of patients admitted to eleven naval hospital ships during that war appears in Appendix F.

In addition to hospital ships and carriers employed by the navy and the army, special provision had to be made for the crews in the convoys of merchant ships which operated throughout the Second World War and which were so frequently under attack from enemy submarines and aircraft.

The inclusion of hospital ships in the convoys was out of the question since Germany seemed to have no intention of honouring the relevant provision of the Geneva convention. Several hospital ships, although clearly marked as such, had been sunk in the first two years of the war (not all of these deliberately, some fell foul of mines).

It was therefore decided that Rescue Ships, manned by Merchant Navy personnel, should accompany the convoys. They were in no way 'Red Cross' ships although many of their duties were similar. They were specially equipped for rescuing survivors from wrecked and blazing ships and had bed accommodation, in tiers, for from 100 to 150 survivors, and mattresses for as many more. Each Rescue Ship had a well-equipped sick bay of six to eight cots and an operating theatre, and their crews included a naval medical officer and one or more sick-berth attendants.

Twenty-nine of these vessels were operational during the war; six were lost at sea. Their full story has been told in *The Rescue Ships* by Schofield and Martyn but the following typifies the rescue work which they undertook.

The *Bury* did exceptionally good work between 11 and 13 May, 1942. Her convoy had been attacked during the night and within three-quarters of an hour she had rescued 45 survivors from one of the torpedoed ships. Fifty minutes later 21 survivors from another torpedoed vessel had been taken on board and then the solitary occupant from a lifeboat was rescued. Later 34 more seamen were taken on board from a Swedish vessel which had been torpedoed twice within 24 hours, and at noon on the 13th 40 survivors from yet another torpedoed ship were rescued. One man died after an operation but five days later the *Bury* reached port with the remaining 177 survivors—her crew strained and exhausted, her supplies reduced to a minimum.

One particularly interesting voyage of the *Stockport* took place in October and November, 1942, when she was homeward bound. Just after midnight one night she rescued the entire crew of a torpedoed vessel and from then on there were a succession of vessels being torpedoed and sinking. Rescue work was slow and the *Stockport* spent many hours cruising to scattered groups of seamen in the water. After she had picked up the survivors from six vessels her propeller was damaged, but rescue work continued and 53 more survivors were taken on board from another vessel. By this time there were 256 survivors and 64 crew on board and the captain was ordered to make for Iceland. After breaking out of the ring of submarines surrounding the main convoy the *Stockport* reached the island. On this voyage alone she covered 5,645 miles, mostly in bitterly cold weather. During the period of her operational duty from 22 October, 1941, this rescue ship saved over 400 lives, but on 24 February, 1943, when searching for survivors from an attacked convoy, she herself was torpedoed and she sank with the loss of 64 crew and 91 survivors of earlier sinkings.

Other ships used for casualties were adapted Landing Ships Tank, Landing Ships Infantry and Motor Fishing vessels. Landing Ships Tank [LST] were fitted with three-tier tubular stretcher racks while additional stretchers could be placed on the tank deck amidships and they were able to take between 300 and 350 stretcher cases, with 160 walking casualties. They carried a medical staff of three naval medical officers (one of whom was a surgeon), 11 Sick-Berth Attendants (including two operating-room attendants) together with 11 seamen ratings and five Royal Marine other ranks to assist the medical orderlies. The vessels were intended to carry casualties for only limited distances and their ability to reach very shallow water made them invaluable in the first assault phases of amphibious operations when only a limited number of hospital carriers were available, and where hospital ships could not be used. During the Normandy invasion some 18,000 casualties were evacuated to the United Kingdom by 70 LST until hospital ships could be employed, and special reception 'hards' were constructed at Gosport, Stokes Bay and Southampton to facilitate the unloading of the vessels.

One of these invaluable vessels was HMLST *363*, which took casualties off the Normandy beaches from D-Day up till the end of June, 1944. She made three journeys across the Channel back to England—the first with 185 casualties (of whom 112 were stretcher cases), the journey taking 32 hours. On the second trip she only carried 96 patients, though again the majority were stretcher cases—this trip was done in 26 hours. On her last journey she took on 279 casualties in exactly two hours—188 were stretcher cases, but as the vessel was only equipped to accommodate 150 on the stretcher racks the other 38 remained lying on the deck on their stretchers. Fortunately on this occasion the journey took only 14 hours. During the three trips 45 operations were performed on board.

In 1944 some Landing Ships Infantry were specially fitted in such a way that as soon as the landing parties had gone ashore the vessel could function as an emergency hospital carrier. Although none were completed in time for use in the European theatre, they did valuable service in the Burma campaign in 1945.

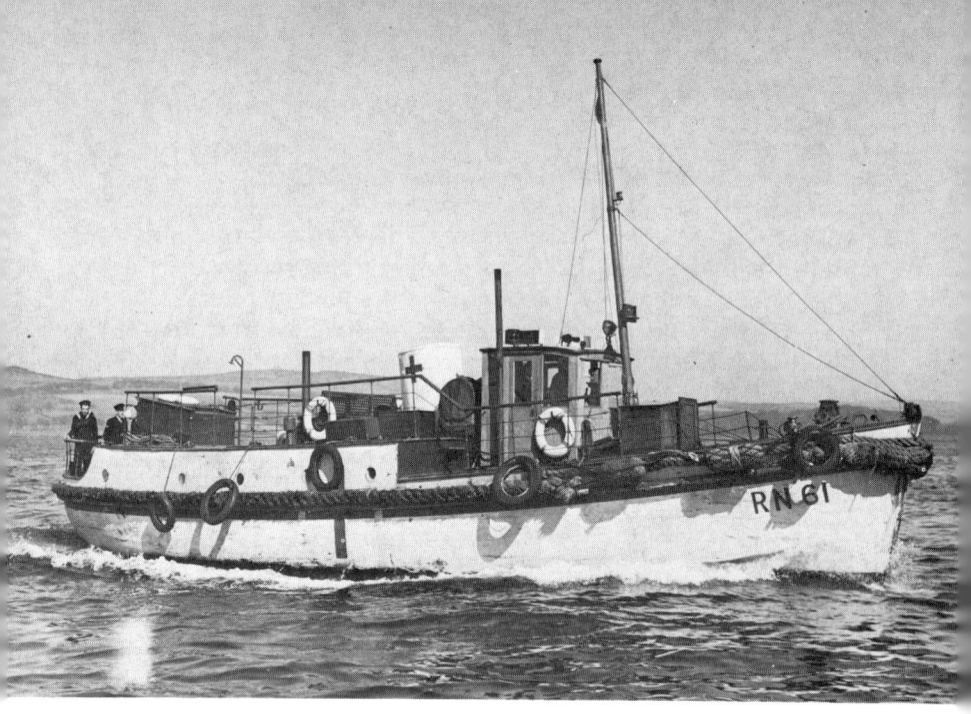

21 One of a number of ferry boats converted to carry casualties to Royal Naval hospital ships

About 50 'medically-fitted' Motor Fishing Vessels were in service during the war. They were adapted to carry 8 to 10 cot cases and from 12 to 20 who could walk, and were particularly used to go alongside ships lying at anchor outside ports and harbours. In addition they frequently transported invalids on coastal routes from one port to another, such as was found necessary in Iceland. Besides doing duty at Scapa Flow, Greenock and the larger ports in the United Kingdom, the MFVs were extensively used during the North African operations and the assaults on Italy. Some went to ports in India and Ceylon and for general service in the South East Asia Command. In December, 1944, four were attached to the British Pacific Fleet for use at Sydney, Brisbane and Freemantle.

The Royal Navy also hired and adapted four 'Hospital Drifters' and three 'Hospital Tenders'.

CHAPTER 5

The Naval Hospital Ship, HMHS Maine

In historical naval tradition, HMHS *Maine* has been perpetuated in a long line of hospital ships. The earliest record of a hospital ship of that name comes from the South African War, when it referred to a vessel given by Bernard H. Baker, then President of the Atlantic Transport Company of Baltimore, New York. Her conversion cost more than £41,000 and was undertaken by a Committee of American ladies in London under the Presidency of Lady Randolph Churchill. Winston Churchill later wrote: 'While I had been busy in South Africa my mother had not been idle at home. She had raised a fund, captivated an American millionaire, obtained a ship, equipped it as a hospital with a full staff of nurses and every comfort', and he noted the coincidence that 'she received her younger son as the very first casualty on board the hospital ship *Maine*'.

The *Maine* was chiefly used as a base military hospital ship at Durban, but during the war she made two trips to England. Then in 1900 she sailed from Southampton to China where she dealt with the sick and wounded of all nationalities during the Boxer Rebellion. She subsequently became a permanent hospital ship of the British fleet and for some years was on service in the Mediterranean, either as a floating hospital or for the transport of naval and military invalids. As the naval hospital ship of the Grand Fleet she was present at the famous Review by His Majesty King George V at Torbay on 27 July, 1910. Her service ended when she ran ashore in thick fog on the Isle of Mull, off the west coast of Scotland on 19 June, 1914. All her patients were safely removed but she had to be abandoned.

The next *Maine* was formerly the *Swansea* and was presented to the Royal Navy on 29 June, 1901, still during the South African War. She was sold on 6 July, 1914, having also stranded.

A third hospital ship named *Maine* had been the *Heliopolis* and was purchased to be a naval hospital ship on 7 March, 1913. She was sold exactly three years later.

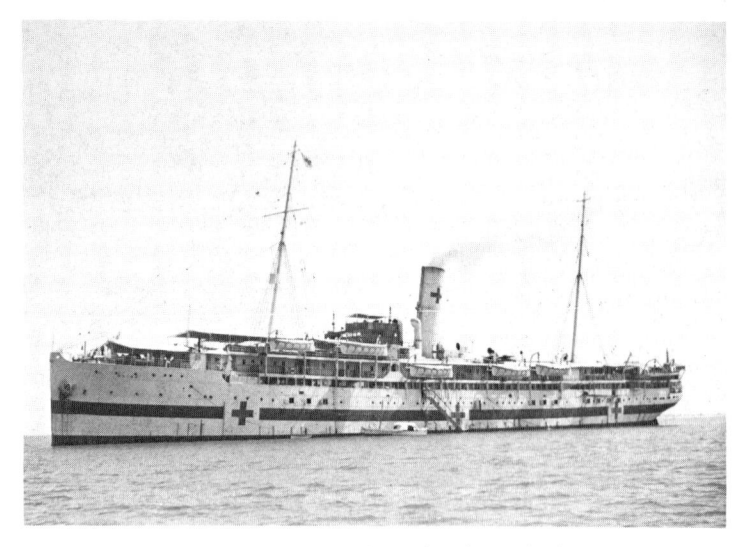

22 The fourth Hospital Ship *Maine*, formerly the *Panama*

The name was again used by the navy in 1920 when the Admiralty purchased the First World War military hospital ship *Panama* and renamed her *Maine*. She was converted for naval use during the following year. The vessel, a coal-burner built in 1902, had a speed of eight to ten knots and was the only hospital ship kept in permanent commission between 1918 and 1939, being placed under the direction of the Commander-in-Chief, Mediterranean Station. Her normal peacetime programme was to accompany the Mediterranean Fleet on its routine cruises, and between such cruises to perform the duties of a base hospital ship for the submarine and destroyer flotillas at Malta. She was occasionally detached for special duties and for some months in 1926 was attached to the China Fleet. In 1935, during the Italian invasion of Abyssinia, she was employed as a base hospital ship at Alexandria for ten months. In September, 1936, the Maine was loaned to the War Office during the Falestine troubles, being based at Haifa. During most of 1937 and 1938 she was employed in the evacuation of refugees between the opposing sides in the Spanish Civil War. By this time the Maine had aged considerably and periodic repairs were no longer able to deal with the ever increasing list of defects. This helped the decision, in 1937, that for the first time the Royal Navy was to have a vessel specially built for hospital ship duties. Plans were completed and approved by April, 1 9 3 9, but the outbreak of the war caused the project to be abandoned. So the old HMHS lWaine had to 'sailor on' throughout the war. At the beginning of 1940 she reached Malta and remained in the Mediterranean for the next two years, for the most part as a base hospital ship at Alexandria. Here, in 1941, she was damaged in an enemy air raid and four members of her crew were killed and twelve injured. Early in 1943 the Maine was lent to the army as a military hospital carrier, in which role she covered a number of North African ports and travelled over 221000 miles, transporting in all more than 6,500 patients. From January to September, 1944, she again did base naval hospital ship duties at Alexandria and then from October to January, 1945, took part in the liberation of Greece. In the latter month she was at Salonika, while the remainder of 1945 was spent at Alexandria and Malta. She reverted to her peacetime naval hospital ship duties at the end of the war. The last reference to this Maine is when she arrived at Bo'ness on 8 July, 1948, to be broken up.

The next, and last, naval hospital ship to carry the name Maine had an interesting background. When taken over by the army she was the Empire Clyde, a government-owned liner managed by the City Line. She had been an Italian ship built in 1925 and named the Leonardo d.a Vincibut had been captured at Massawa and converted into a military hospital ship with 411 beds. The Admiralty used the Ernpire Clyde in May, 1945, as one of the additional naval hospital ships that were then required for the British Pacific Fleet. Her first journey from the

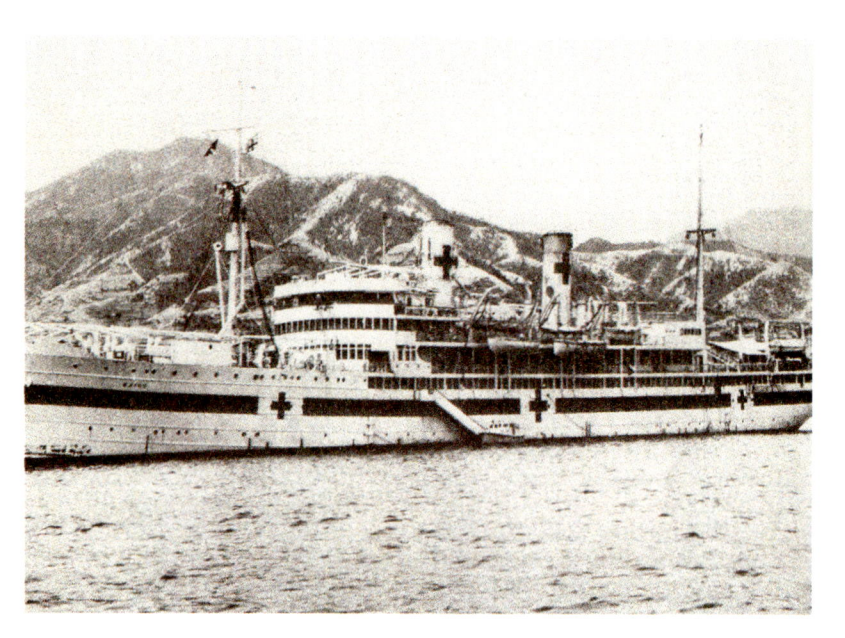

23 The last HMHS Maine, the only naval hospital ship to be awarded a battle honour:'Korea 1950'

United Kingdom to the Far East was on 28 July, 1945. During the remainder of that year and in 1946 she was on service at Manus, Shanghai, Singapore and Hong Kong--{oing a long spell at Hong Kong as base hospitd ship. The Empire Clyde was then permanently taken over from the Ministry of Transport as a naval hospital ship and renamed HMHS Iulaine, replacing the one broken up at Bo'ness. Her final operational commission was during the Korean War in 1950-1953 when she was placed at the disposal of the United Nations Forces. Staffed by Royal Naval Medical Service personnel she was extensively used for ferrying UN casualties, mostly American, from Korea to US army base hospitals in Japan. At that time her accommodation consisted of two decks of wards--an upper level comprising 116 beds in five wards, while the lower level (also divided into five wards) had 156 double-tiered beds. There was also an officers'ward of 16 beds on the upper deck. Among the many medical and surgical facilities were an air-conditioned major operating theatre, an X-Ray room, a dispensary and a surgery. HMHS Maine ended her operational service in Hong Kong on 26 Aprtl,1954, where she was sold & where, it is believed, she was broken up.
PAGE 70.

The project to give the Royal Navy a specially-built hospital ship—abandoned on the outbreak of the Second World War—was reconsidered in the 1950s and a ship of 10,000 tons, to be called HMHS *Maine,* was laid down in the yard of Barclay Curle in 1952. But once again the project was cancelled. Nevertheless, the most famous name among Royal Navy hospital ships has a permanent tribute, for the last HMHS *Maine* was one of the British ships awarded the Battle Honour 'Korea 1950'. The list of awards of naval battle honours is distinguished and goes back from the Korean War over 385 years to the Spanish Armada. Of the more than 780 ships listed, there is only one hospital ship: 'HMHS *Maine*—Korea—1950'.

CHAPTER 6

Hospital Ships for Merchant Seamen and Deep-Sea Fishermen

This chapter tells the story of the use of ships for the hospital and medical needs of merchant seamen and deep-sea fishermen, and it starts in the early 1800's when cholera reached Sunderland and London from the Baltic. In one year there were nearly 15,000 cases and a third of them proved fatal. The disease particularly attacked the merchant seamen of Britain who had played such a part in saving the nation from defeat during the naval blockade of the Napoleonic wars. The seamen's plight was made yet more pathetic since the benefits of Greenwich Hospital (which was used for patients from the Royal Navy) were not available to them.

On 8 March, 1821, a Seamen's Hospital Society was formed, and in that year the *Grampus,* a former 48-gun ship, was loaned by the Admiralty for conversion into a hospital ship. On 19 October, 1821, she was victualled by the Society and provided with bedding and linen from the Royal Naval Hospital at Haslar. She was then moored off Greenwich to receive sick seamen off ships passing upstream, the first being taken on board on 25 October. The staff and crew of the *Grampus* comprised a Superintendant, a surgeon, a steward and clerk, a boatswain and carpenter, two boatswain's mates, three male nurses, a male cook, and a washerwoman. The wards were on the lower decks and were lit by whale-oil lamps, while operations on patients sometimes had to be performed by candlelight. By the end of the year 431 merchant seamen patients had spent some time in the *Grampus.*

The work of the Seamen's Hospital so impressed the Board of Admiralty that on 27 September, 1822, the Lords Commissioners issued a special Warrant authorizing the *Grampus* to wear the Jack and Pendant of the Sovereign's Ships—usually a jealously guarded prerogative of the Royal Navy.

Ten years later, by which time the *Grampus* was too small for the work she had to do, the Admiralty agreed that she should be replaced by a larger hulk, the *Dreadnought*, a '98-gun 1st rate' which had fought at Trafalgar and had previously been used by the Royal Navy as a hospital ship at Milford Haven. The *Dreadnought*, which could accommodate 250 patients and 150 convalescents, was in use from 31 October, 1831, until 25 January, 1857.

Cholera was common in the earlier years of the century and hospital ships were largely maintained as isolation vessels. By 1832 the situation had grown so serious that HMS *Dover* was fitted up for the reception of 200 seamen and sent to join the *Dreadnought* and the *Iphigenia* at Greenwich. At the same time another ship, HMS *Tremendous*, was being prepared for the reception of naval ratings, but by the time she was ready the outbreak was on the decline.

In 1835 the Seamen's Hospital Society took over HMS *Dover*, *Devonshire* and *Belleisle*, as well as other ships to combat a further outbreak of the disease.

By 1856 the *Dreadnought* in turn proved too small to accommodate the numbers of seamen requiring treatment, and on 26 January, 1857, she was replaced at Greenwich by HMS *Caledonia*, a 120-gun ship and the former flagship of Lord Exmouth. When she came into service as a hospital, *Caledonia's* name was changed to *Dreadnought*.

In the 1860's the question arose as to whether the *Dreadnought* should move or a new hospital be built ashore. The result was that on 13 April, 1870, the seamen patients were moved from the ship into the Infirmary at Greenwich which, together with the Somerset Ward, was leased by the Admiralty to the Seamen's Hospital Society at one shilling per annum. The *Dreadnought*, however, remained at Grenwich for a further two years as isolation accommodation but departed from her moorings in 1872, thus ending an epoch in the history of the present Dreadnought Seamen's Hospital at Greenwich.

The fishermen of the North Sea were in need of hospital

ships as much as the merchant seamen, and this responsibility was accepted by the National Mission to Deep Sea Fishermen (NMDSF) which was founded by E. J. Mather in 1881, apparently having originated from the Thames Church Mission. The Mission initially administered only to the spiritual needs of the North Sea fishermen, later extending its service to those fishing the south and west coasts of Ireland and subsequently to the cod fishermen of Newfoundland and Labrador.

There were always many injuries and illnesses among fishermen. The job was, and still is, one of the most hazardous and uncomfortable of all. They worked in cramped conditions in small vessels, usually in rough seas and often in temperatures below freezing. Any treatment received on board was given by the skipper from the ship's 'dispensary' which contained mixtures, pills, ointments, a 'surgical chest' and other items. At first these facilities were most elementary, but later were greatly improved when Dr A. Schofield, an 'Honorary Physician and Surgical Instructor', trained skippers in the 'principles of surgery and medicine' with the result that many obtained certificates, either of the St John Ambulance Brigade or of the National Health Society. But even after they had been treated by their modestly-qualified skippers the patients had to make the 300–350 mile trip back to the Thames on one of the catch carriers for admission to the London Hospital which served London's dockland.

Mr Mather, who was chiefly interested in the spiritual salvation of fishermen, soon realized that physical rescues were frequently as necessary, and that it was important that treatment should be given on the spot. The Mission therefore decided that vessels with doctors should be able to attend the fishing fleets, and the first to do so was the *Ensign*. This vessel, which cost over £1,000, was provided with a large ship's medicine chest containing medicines, simple surgical instruments, ointments, bandages and splints, together with manuals of treatment. She made her first trip in July, 1882, and when she reached the fishing fleet immediately dealt with some members of the crews of ten trawlers. Such was the inauguration of the hospital ship activties of the present Royal National Mission to Deep Sea Fishermen.

In 1886 Dr Frederick Treves, who later earned professional fame and a knighthood after performing an appendectomy on King Edward VII, was elected a Member of the Mission and became Chairman of the Medical Department. He envisaged a fuller medical service for fishermen, with vessels equipped as 'floating hospitals'. The immediate outcome was the appearance of the Mission ship Clulow which was authorized to be used as a hospital ship for a period of two months. Dr Wilfred Thomason Grenfell volunteered to serve on the Clulow, was accepted by Dr Treves, and in December, 1888, was appointed the Mission's doctor at a salary of {300 ayear. By the end of the following year he had become the Mission's Medical Superintendent; with his strong evangelical feelings he was as much interested in the spiritual as in the medical needs of the fishermen.

At the time of the formation of the NMDSF there were about 200 tanned-sail smacks of 50 to 80 tons fishing in huge fleets on the Dogger Bank in the North Sea, between 54" and 56'North latitude. Each carried a crew of four or more and each fleet was accompanied by carriers which collected the catch and took it to the home ports while the trawlers continued fishing. Thus there could be at anv one time some thousands of fishermen in a more or less confined area-a factor which made it paratively easy for the Mission's vessels to carry out duties.

In 1886 the Mission also became aware of the medical needs of the cod fishermen across the Atlantic but it did not become actively involved until 1891 when Mr Francis Hopwood (later Lord Southborough) a member of the Mission Council, went to Canada in his capacity as an official of the Board of Trade. He stayed at St John's, Newfoundland, for a week and on his return home wrote a lengthy report describing the plight of the fishermen, not only there but dso off Labrador.

Then, in 1892, 40 out of 200 fishermen working from Trinity Bay, East Newfoundland, were lost In a storm at sea and the Lord Mayor of London launched an appeal to help their families. As a result of this publicity the Mission received many requests for practical help, and it was decided to send a 'hospital ship' on an exploratory voyage. The vessel selected

was the Albert, which was authorized to make a voyage from Yarmouth to St John's, cruise the Newfoundland and Labrador coastq call at any port between 40o and 60o North, and return to the United Kingdom within two years. Carrying a master, a mate, a crew of seven and with Dr Grenfell as the surgeon, she left the River Yare on 12 June, 1892, and reached St John's on 22luly.

When the Albert arrived at St John's the town was in ruins, as more than 2,000 buildings--the former homes of the entire population of some 11,000-had been destroyed by fire, fortunately without loss of life. The Albert remained at the devastated port for about five weeks, Dr Grenfell giving medical aid to all who needed it. She left for Labrador on 2 August, sailed as far north as Hopedale (about 1,000 miles away), cruised the Belle Isle Strait, and altogether dedt with over 900 patients during the 3,000 mile voyaEle.T he voyage, which cost over f,2,000, clearly showed the need for a smaller vessel to operate in the inshore waters of the extensive coast line, and consequently the Princess May, a small steam launch of 45 ft, was shipped to Newfoundland. In this small vessel Dr Grenfell's cabin was used as the hospital.

The voyage of the Albert had emphasized that conditions around Newfoundland and Labrador were very different from those in the North Sea. In the North Sea the fishermen worked from a small number of 'fishing ports'in England and Scotland, and congregated in huge fleets, fishing comparatively confined areas which were rarely further than 350 miles from home. In Newfoundland and Labrador, however, there were thousands of miles of coastline dong which were scattered fishermen of differing nationalities. Those in Newfoundland were English, Scotch, or Irish, with smaller numbers of French descent; in Labrador they were mostly Eskimos, together with some Indians, a number of half-breeds and a number of immigrants from Devon and Cornwall who called themselves'Liveyers' ('the people who live here').

In the many small ports of Newfoundland some 350 vessels v/ere manned by upwards of 4,500 fishermen, while as many as 33,000 sailed from St John's to Labrador where they were joined by about 3,300'Liveyers', who came from their winter

quarters high in the inlets which indent the coast. Medical problems for the fishermen and their families were particularly acute, for there were neither doctors nor hospitals. The Mission therefore not only provided the doctors but also built hospitals, three in Labrador and one in Newfoundland. The Mission vessels with doctors, nurses and medical supplies on board were mainly used as the medical bases where patients could be cared for until periodic visits were made to the various hospitals.

Meanwhile there were continuing improvements made for the fishermen of the North Sea. Another Mission hospital ship, the *Queen Victoria*, went to sea for periods of up to eight weeks at a time, carrying a skipper, a crew of seven or eight and a doctor. The *Queen Victoria* had large airy hospital accommodation amidships with ten berths, two of which were slung and invaluable for fracture cases. Casualties from the fishing fleets could therefore be properly treated on board, and kept under proper medical supervision until the vessel returned to England when, if necessary, they were transferred to hospital. Other Mission hospital ships built during this early period were the *Alice Fisher* (1891), *Alpha* (1899), *Queen Alexandra* (1901) and the *Joseph and Sarah Miles* (1902).

While conditions for the British fishermen had greatly improved, by the late 1890s Dr Grenfell realized that the fishing vessels adapted for hospital duties did not fulfil the requirements of Newfoundland and Labrador. He wanted a 'real' hospital ship and set himself the task of raising funds to buy one. The outcome was the Mission hospital ship *Strathcona*, which was given by Lord Strathcona, Lord Commissioner of Canada. Her keel had been laid down at Dartmouth in 1895 and she was subsequently fitted out as a hospital ship at Yarmouth where her steel hull was reinforced to withstand ice pressure. Like the *Queen Victoria*, the *Strathcona*'s hospital accommodation was amidships and two of her six cots were slung. In addition she had a dispensary, X-ray equipment, electric light, a bathroom, and a wireless set which was given by Marconi himself. In 1898 the *Strathcona* sailed for Newfoundland and Dr Grenfell joined her at Battle Harbour. She remained on duty for over 20 years, until in 1922 her career ended when she ran into a north-west wind in Bonavista Bay, heaved over and sank. Her successor, the *Strathcona II*, was purchased in 1924, and during the following year was reconditioned and fitted-out, at a cost of over £3,000; she served as a Mission hospital ship sailing from Labrador from 1925 until 1959.

By the turn of the century the hospital service of the NMDSF had become fully established; it had more than proved its worth during the 'Dogger Bank Incident' in 1904 during the Russo-Japanese War. The Russian Baltic Squadron, while crossing the North Sea on its way to the Far East, opened fire on a fleet of 50 Hull fishing trawlers fishing on the Dogger Bank on 22 October, 1904. The Russian explanation was that they had been mistaken for Japanese torpedo boats. One trawler, the *Crane*, was sunk, two others, the *Moulmein* and the *Mina*, were damaged, while two fishermen were killed and six wounded, the latter being taken on board the *Alpha* and the *Joseph and Sarah Miles*. The Russians had to pay compensation for this action amounting to some £100,000.

A further indication of the contribution made by the Mission is the fact that in 1910 alone more than 15,000 patients were treated by the Mission's doctors. During the First World War the RNMDSF worked in close association with the Admiralty and one of their smacks went to Scapa Flow where she was converted into a hospital ship to serve as a Mission vessel with the Royal Navy.

In Newfoundland and Labrador, however, the aims of the RNMDSF were being pursued with unflagging energy by Dr Grenfell, so much so that by 1907 various 'Grenfell Associations' had been formed. Financial help for the Mission's work in those areas came increasingly from Canada and the United States of America, and this resulted in the formation in 1925 of the 'International Grenfell Association' (IGA) with Dr Grenfell as President. (He received a knighthood in 1928.) The three hospitals in Labrador and the one in Newfoundland were eventually handed over to the IGA by the RNMDSF, followed in 1959 by the hospital ship *Strathcona II*. Both organizations are still in existence and although the IGA is based at St John's, Newfoundland, its affairs are conducted from Boston and New

York. As late as 1959 the Association had two hospital ships, both operating from St Anthony, Newfoundland.

The Mission hospital ship *Albert* entered service off Newfoundland and Labrador largely as a result of the shock caused by the loss of 40 fishermen in the area. History has a habit of repeating itself and it did so as recently as the severe winter of 1967–1968 when altogether 5 British trawlers were lost in the Icelandic fishing grounds with a death toll of 59 fishermen. The Government took action and the Board of Trade chartered the *Orsino*, a modern steam trawler and she was used as a support ship for two winters. Initially her duties were to give weather advice and to provide an experimental medical service, the latter being undertaken by four doctors working in six-week spells. Because she was a working trawler her hospital accommodation was quite small and was in two sections. The surgery was a fairly large cabin stripped of bunks and given a couch, desk, medical locker, sink, sterilizer, water heater and additional heating and lighting; the hospital section was a smaller cabin fitted with a double-tier hospital cot. The *Orsino* spent the winters of 1968–1969 and 1969–1970 on patrol and the doctors (in the second winter assisted by a sick berth attendant) treated 178 patients from the small trawlers, as well as numerous members of the crew of the *Orsino* itself. During the second season there were at least 70 radio consultations.

In 1970 the *Orsino* was replaced by the *Miranda*, which did duty with the fishing fleet during the 'Icelandic Cod War' of 1973 and is still on service. She was originally a four-masted schooner called the *Albatross* and was built in 1942 for Swedish sea cadets. Later as the *Donna* (and still under sail) she was strengthened and worked as an ice-breaker in the Antarctic. She was converted into a motor ship in 1967, and in the following year purchased at a cost of £90,000 by the British Government. The *Miranda*'s hospital accommodation includes a ward with two double and two single cots, one of the latter being a 'swinging' cot; there is also a small separate ward with only one cot. The surgery has an operating table (which can be converted into a dental chair) and X-ray apparatus, while the dispensary contains a medical locker, refrigerator, gas cylinders and medical stores.

CHAPTER 7

The Beginning of Railway Ambulance Transport

The passenger railway era may be regarded as having started on 27 September, 1825, when Stephenson's steam engine *Locomotion* hauled a miscellaneous collection of open wagons (many carrying passengers) and a solitary passenger coach on the Stockton and Darlington Railway, in the County of Durham. But the first railway in Britain to carry fare-paying passengers in trains drawn by steam locomotives seems to have been the Canterbury and Whitstabie Railway, which was opened on 3 May, 1830 and inaugurated a passenger service the following day.

Later that year, on 15 September, the Liverpool and Manchester Railway opened a route 30 miles long, this service boasting the first specially designed passenger carriages.

Railways were rapidly laid down in many parts of the world—America being the first to follow Britain in 1830. (Ten years later America had over 3,300 miles of track.) Of the European countries France, in 1832, was first followed by Belgium and Germany in 1835, Austria in 1836, Russia a year later, Italy in 1839, Switzerland in 1844, Poland in the following year, and Denmark and Hungary in 1847.

It is easy to see that strategic considerations were of great importance in the early days of railway construction, especially on the Continent, for no other form of transport could carry troops to frontiers as quickly as a railway. The carriage of casualties on return journeys from the fighting line was an obvious step, and so the use of railway ambulance transport received special consideration from 1859 onwards, during the frequent campaigns and skirmishes in Europe.

With the knowledge of the varying dates on which different countries laid down their railway systems, it is relevant to look at the railway systems as they existed in 1850. With over 9,000 miles, America had pressed furthest ahead, Britain coming next with about 6,500 miles. Germany had 3,700 miles of track and France about 2,000. Belgium had only 560 miles while Austria, Hungary and Italy each had less than 400. These rates of development had considerable effect on the dates on which the countries considered varying kinds of railway ambulance transport systems, for the use of railways for ambulance purposes covers a period of over 120 years from the Crimean War of 1854 to the present.

One famous incident, however, deserves to qualify as the very first occasion on which railway was used as a means of ambulance transport. On 15 September, 1830, William Huskisson, Member of Parliament for Liverpool, had been watching a demonstration of Stephenson's *Rocket*. His attention was distracted during its run, and oblivious of the engineers' warning cries, Huskisson was struck by the *Rocket*. Seriously injured, he was transported on the locomotive *Northumbrian* to Liverpool, but in spite of this rapid means of ambulance transport he died.

The earliest recorded occasion on which a railway was used to convey sick and wounded troops from the battle front was in the Crimean War. The illustration on page 82 is of the commencement of the railway works at Balaklava. This, the first military railway, was seven to eight miles long, had a gauge of 5 ft 3 ins and was specially constructed for the campaign. Store wagons or 'contractors' trucks' carried supplies to the troops on the line between Balaklava and Sevastopol. At first they were drawn by horses and mules—stationary engines being used at steep places. They were subsequently powered by steam railway locomotives, two of which were named *Alliance* and *Victory*. (Before the railway was built some 2,000 horses had been used to move the 112 tons of supplies needed at the camp each day.) With the advent of the railway, the empty wagons were used on the return journey to evacuate casualties from the camp hospitals in the forward areas to hospitals in the rear—but at first only sitting cases were carried.

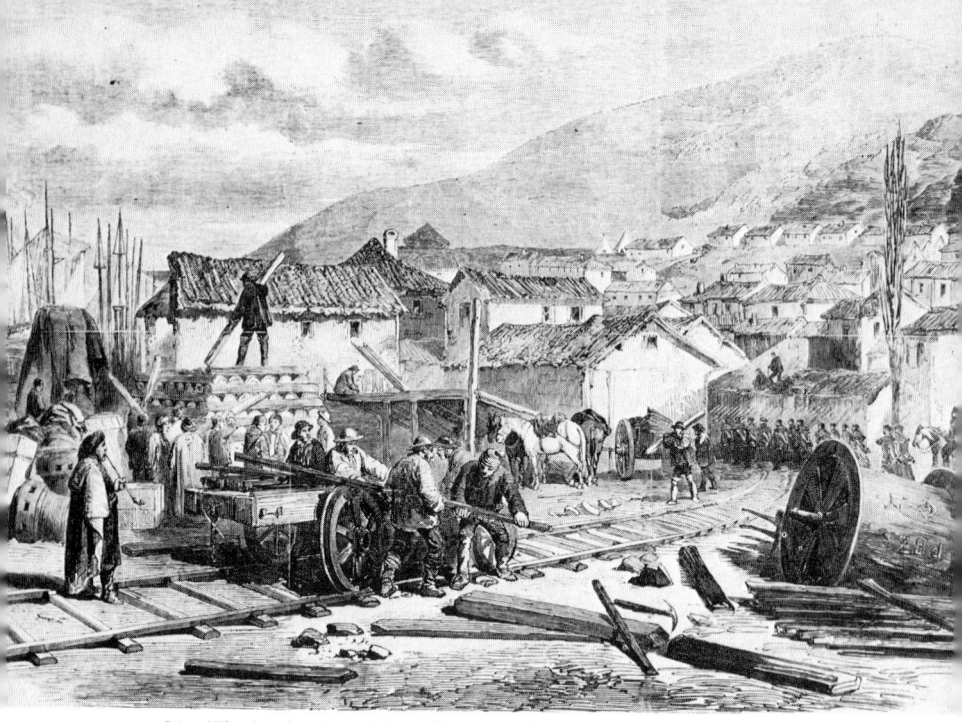

24 The beginning of the railway works at Balaklava; contractors' trucks carried stores to the forward areas and brought back sick and wounded on the return journey

The Crimean War was also a landmark in British military medical history in two other respects. It was the first occasion on which an ambulance transport service manned by British troops was used—the Hospital Conveyance Corps having been raised on 4 May, 1854. (This had a very brief existence, being incorporated in the Land Transport Corps on 21 July, 1855.) But much more important was the appearance of Florence Nightingale—that legendary figure of the Crimean War who organized a band of nurses, and did such great service in relieving the sufferings of the sick and wounded troops. Her actions led to the creation of the Army Nursing Service, whose history has led it from poke bonnets and long, voluminous skirts to steel helmets and regulation battle dress.

These innovations in medical treatment were firmly established, and railway ambulance transport was, after the Crimean War, used extensively on the Continent. A 'railway sick transport carriage', constructed out of an ordinary wagon, was used by the French at Châlons in 1857. Railway ambulance transport was used in the Italian–Austrian War of 1859, the Schleswig–Holstein War of 1864, the Austro–Prussian–Italian conflict of 1866, the Franco–German War of 1870–1871 and the Servian–Bulgarian War of 1885–1886. It was also extensively used in the American Civil War of 1861–1864, by Britain in the Zulu War of 1879 and during the Boer rebellion in 1881, in the Egyptian campaigns of 1884 and 1885, the rebellion in Rhodesia in 1896, and in the Sudan campaign of 1898. Patients were carried in railway vehicles in the Turco–Greek war of 1897, the Russo–Japanese War of 1904, in the Balkan War of 1912–1913, and by both sides in the South African War of 1899–1902. All participants in the two world wars made considerable use of modern ambulance trains which were constantly being brought up-to-date.

Initially, of course, the systems were extremely primitive, such as in the 1859 Italian–Austrian campaign, when railway ambulance transport was used by both sides. In some cases even seriously wounded soldiers were laid on straw in cattle trucks—at other times travelling in ordinary passenger carriages. At one stage over 1,000 casualties a night travelled from Brescia to Milan and the patients suffered considerably on these journeys; altogether about 89,000 casualties were carried by railway in this war.

More serious consideration of the use of railway transport for the movement of sick and wounded was instigated in Prussia in 1860 by the Prussian War Minister, Von Roon, who made experiments to ascertain the best methods to be used. Up to this time the majority of patients still travelled in wagons which only had a floor covering of straw. Subsequently they were carried on suspended stretchers which were supported by straps, buckles and rubber rings. The less seriously wounded continued to travel in various classes of passenger coaches and carriages. When railway vehicles were used solely for ambulance purposes in the Italian–Austrian War, a doctor and an attendant, together with a supply of medicine and medical equipment also travelled on the train. During this period another experiment in comfort was tried—sacks of straw which had three canvas loops on each side into which poles could be inserted, thus converting the sack into a stretcher.

It was as a result of these experiments that Dr Gurlt, a German, introduced the *paillasse* method which was simply filling mattress covers with straw and laying patients on them on the floors of the various railway vehicles. He had previously suggested that hammocks should be suspended from the roofs of the vans. But the roofs sometimes collapsed under the weight of the occupied hammocks, which anyway swung with the motion of the train and resulted in the patients hitting the sides of the railway vehicles.

When the American Civil War started on 12 May, 1861, there were just over 30,000 miles of railways in that country, mostly of single track, with gauges varying from 6 ft to 4 ft 9 ins, while some were even narrower. Nevertheless some or all of these railways systems appear to have been used for the transport of casualties on both sides. In 1862 some wounded troops were unloaded from trains at Atlanta (originally called Terminus) which was a junction of four railway systems—one running to the west, another to the south, a third to the coast and the other via Augusta towards the north and east. By 1864 train-loads of patients were flooding through Atlanta.

Large numbers of casualties were carried from the fighting area by ordinary passenger carriages, improvised goods wagons, or specially fitted transport cars. The latter were adapted to carry 24 stretchers per car (12 on either side), suspended from wooden supports by rubber rings. Normally each of the cars had an iron stove in the centre and they were coupled to ordinary passenger trains.

After the Battle of Gettysburg about 15,000 patients were moved by railway to Baltimore, Harrisburg, Philadelphia and York, many lying on straw in freight cars. Usually 20 stretchers were crowded into the limited spaces and ventilation was provided by cutting holes in the sides and ends of the wagons.

Between the morning of 12 June and the evening of 14 June, 1863, nearly 10,000 victims of the Federal disaster at Chancellorsville were carried by the Aquita Creek railway to Washington. In that year sick and wounded were frequently transported in wagons which had rows of one or two tiers of wooden bunks supported on upright posts. Later on rubber rings were fitted to the post, into which the handles of stretchers could be inserted.

Earlier on, in 1862, the Philadelphia Railroad Company had

adapted a sleeping car for railway ambulance work with its supports arranged so that stretcher cases could easily be moved in and out, though a drawback was the lack of uniformity of the stretchers used. These wagons accommodated 50 patients, and were fitted with a seat for an orderly at each end of the car, a stove, water-tank and a locker.

On another occasion 1,500 casualties made a 50-mile journey travelling in goods wagons from Olustee to Jacksonville on the Mobile Railway, in this case the floors being strewn with a little straw plus a few branches of pine.

It was during the Civil War that complete, yet improvised ambulance trains appear to have first been used. Their formation was ordered by the Medical Director of the Department at Washington, and they were made up of nine or ten ward-cars for patients, with separate wagons for cooking, stores, and as a dispensary. There was also accommodation provided for the staff.

On 11 August, 1863, the Medical Officer of the Army of the Cumberland was instructed to fit up a special train for hospital purposes to run between Nashville, Tennessee and Louisville; it was to be made up of the best rolling stock in use and of new cars. By 1864 three such trains were running regularly—each covering a section of the 472 mile track between Atlanta and Louisville. The trains (carrying 175–200 patients) had five large, open 'American' passenger cars as ward-cars for cot cases, and another car for sitting patients. There were also cars for the staff, for use as a kitchen, another which was a dispensary, and a conductor's car. (The total casualties evacuated from the advanced lines at Nashville and Louisville has been given as 20,000. Taking the American Civil War as a whole, the number of troops on both sides who were killed, wounded or who died of wounds has been estimated at over half a million.)

A year after the American Civil War ended in 1865, hospital trains in Europe were as unsophisticated as they had been in America before the war. During the Battle of Sadowa, when the Prussians won a decisive victory over the Austrians on the upper Elbe, casualties were taken in ordinary passenger coaches and in goods wagons to Dresden and Prague. The journey must have been extremely uncomfortable; it lasted up to two days, and there was no medical attention for the casualties.

After the end of the Prussian–Italian War of 1866 a Prussian commission of military and medical authorities investigated the carriage of sick and wounded by rail transport. At the end of three months they decided against the American system of rubber-ringed suspended stretchers, opting instead for straw-filled paillasses, and claiming that patients would feel uncomfortable if carried one above the other! The Commission recommended the adaption of fourth class coaches as 'vestibule trains' so that not only could the doctors and the staff move throughout the train while it was travelling, but also that medical supplies and cooking facilities would be available to all.

The findings of the Prussian Commission were largely responsible for a series of experiments carried out at the 1867 Paris *Exposition Internationale,* under the direction of some of the International Committee of Delegates, formed from Societies for Aid to Wounded in Time of War. The *Chemin de Fer de l'Ouest* supplied a short length of track and a goods van, in which a number of systems were tried out, using a considerable variety of fittings.

Transport contrivances for the sick were collected from various countries—the chief ones being exhibited by the Baden Committee. Among the appliances exhibited was a Dr Gauvin's spring stretcher, eight of which could be contained in a goods wagon; a model of one of the American coaches, fitted with rubber rings for carrying stretchers, was also there. Some of the many appliances and contrivances for the railway transport of sick and wounded were subsequently included in the Museum of Military Surgery at the Royal Victoria Hospital, Netley. Among them was a portable mattress for use in a first-class carriage—just one mattress to one carriage!

Baron Mundy, who had had some experience of the use of trains carrying sick and wounded in the Austrian war of 1866, attended the Exposition. Dr Gurlt, who had introduced the paillasse system, was also there. Mundy, however, favoured covering the floors of railway vehicles with considerable quantities of straw first, and then laying down the filled paillasses. This was found to reduce jolting considerably and thus avoid much of the discomfort.

In Berlin in the same year a plan for the conveyance of the severely wounded was made applicable to all railway systems in the North German Confederation. Fourth class carriages were adapted for this purpose and entrances were made at each end. Alterations were also made to the interiors of the carriages, so that each could carry twelve patients on stretchers which were suspended on wooden supports. With the adoption of this plan and with customary German efficiency, all fourth class carriages of these railway systems were from then on constructed with doors at each end. Prussian goods wagons were at that time also adapted to carry twelve stretcher cases each, using a similar support system.

The 1867 trials in Paris led to renewed interest in the question of the carriage of sick and wounded by rail transport; another Prussian Commission on the subject was appointed, and there was a serious discussion at the International Congress of Red Cross Societies in 1869. As a result of the findings of the second Commission, the Prussian government adopted a 'standard' system—which was mainly used in the Franco–Prussian War of 1870–1871, when the Prussians had an admirable service for the evacuation of their sick and wounded by rail transport.

They had twenty-one 'sanitary' trains in use, all of which were adapted from rolling stock by the use of the 'Grund' system. Separate coaches carried lying and sitting patients, while the personnel had coaches of their own. Other coaches were used for the carriage of provisions, water, fuel and baggage. The trains accommodated varying numbers of patients (the maximum being 149 lying and 220 sitting) but despite the relatively high standard of accommodation, discomfort did not cease with boarding the train; in one case, for instance, it took eight days for a train to go from Gomeru, just outside Paris, to Berlin, while in November, 1871, the sick and wounded who entrained at Lagny in open trucks spent five to eight days travelling to Germany, during which time they were unable to leave their trucks, and the only available provisions were biscuits or dry bread, and possibly a drink of water. Nevertheless, approximately 90,000 casualties were transported by train during this war.

In the Russo-Turkish War of 1877–1878 approximately 188,000 patients were transported by train. On 23 December, 1877, 600 Turkish casualties arrived at Bucharest in a 'hospital' train made up of vans rather like horse-boxes. The patients were in a deplorable condition, having been delayed on the journey by intense cold and were off-loaded into carts and taken to hospital. On the last day of that year 64 Turkish patients, more comfortably accommodated, were taken by train to Varna.

In the Servian–Bulgarian War of 1885–1886 Major-General Laurie from England worked with Baron Mundy in fitting out a hospital train composed of passenger coaches which had been cleared of seats and fitted with slings to take stretchers. The train, which was provided by the British Red Cross Society and the Austrian Maltese Order, left Belgrade on 31 December, 1885, detrained convalescent soldiers at almost every station along the line, and reached Nis at 11 am the next day, having carried 152 patients during the journey.

In India, during the peaceful years of the 1880's, troops arriving at Bombay from the United Kingdom rested for a few days at Deolali. They then travelled in special trains, each of which included a second-class carriage which had six sleeping berths in one half, the other half being occupied by an apothecary. When a number of invalids had to be carried, first class compartments were converted by the use of the 'Zavodovski' system of improvisation, which enabled each to hold from eight to twelve beds. In addition there was a special train in which a 'Collis dandy' was used—a bamboo-frame stretcher-like apparatus supported on bamboo legs. Twelve patients could be carried in each carriage of this special train. These systems of improvisation, most of which converted large postal, goods, fruit, fish and similar trucks, vans and wagons had one idea in common—the carriage of patients in a railway vehicle, on stretchers, with the least amount of discomfort. In some cases the handles of stretchers were placed in loops in ropes, sometimes one above the other, the ropes being suspended from the roof of the vehicles. In others blocks of wood were fixed to the sides of the vans with a rounded notch to take the inner handle of the stretcher while the outer handle was supported by straps hanging from the ceilings. In other cases metal fitments were fastened in the vans and the stretchers carried on frames. These systems were the invention of Austrian, Bavarian, French, German, Russian and other Europeans as will be seen from the following list of names of the systems—Austrian; Berlin; Boulomie; Bréchot-Déspres-Amelines; Compt de Beaufort; Gurley; Grund; Hamburg; Heidelberg; Linxweiler; Morache; Ponts and Zavodovski.

The Zavodovski method was invented by a Russian engineer and Major-General of that name in 1873; it was used by the British in India and details of it were included in the *Manual of Medical Staff Corps*, 1893, and in *Royal Army Medical Corps Training*, 1911, which lists the apparatus required for one coach, as 4 cables 9 ft long and over 1 in thick, ringed at each end, the inner portion of the ring strengthened by a metal collar-shaped band; 16 stout looped ropes (the thickness of a drag-rope) tied in the centre so as to support the upper tier of stretchers; 8 large iron hooks; 32 small ring-bolts; 4 solid circular poles, 6 ft long and 2 in thick; 8 stretchers (army pattern) and 28 stout cords for lashings.

It was the Bréchot-Déspres-Amelines system which was selected by the British Army Medical authorities as being the most suitable for use in war. The apparatus was therefore included in the mobilization equipment for the medical services and was available for immediate use on the outbreak of the First World War, being extensively used in the early phases of the war.

One of the very early specially constructed hospital trains was the Sanitary Train of the *Société Francaise*. There were separate wagons for four surgeons, with others for the carriage of stores, for use as a kitchen and one, the last in the train, being a magazine. Twenty wagons, fitted with connecting doors, were used for patients and the train accommodated 300 lying and 500 sitting patients.

A much more elaborate train was that of the 'Knights of Malta and the Grand Priory of Bohemia'. There were then separate carriages for the Commandant and for the medical officers, and a dining wagon for the other members of the staff. One carriage was used for provisions, another as a kitchen and a separate one for general stores. This train only accommodated 100 lying patients, however, ten in each of ten carriages. The Inventory of the train helps to explain its low carrying capacity. It listed more than 100 items—including glasses for champagne, port, claret, sherry, wine and liqueurs, as well as wine decanters and beer tumblers, spoons and nut crackers. As only a few of each of these items were carried, they were obviously for the use of the staff of the train! But there were also considerable numbers of knives, forks and spoons of various descriptions on the inventory—together with 1,000 tooth-picks, so the patients were not entirely forgotten.

Other trains were equipped by the Austro-Hungarian National Red Cross Society and were held in readiness at Vienna—the government providing them with personnel.

Another attempt to produce a hospital train of a comfortable, almost luxurious construction, was made in the 1870's, and was exhibited at the Great Paris exhibitions. But, as stated earlier, it is likely that America was the first to have a practical, properly designed hospital train, during the American Civil War in 1862.

In England in 1870 Surgeon-General Sir T. Longmore drew up a plan for a carriage to transport patients by rail from Portsmouth to Netley. One was constructed at the Metropolitan works at Birmingham; it had a side entrance as well as folding doors at each end, and contained eight bunks—four on either side—on which patients on stretchers were placed. There was a seat for the medical officer, under which were lockers for medicines and other supplies, and hinged seats for the orderlies. This carriage also had a stove, a water-closet with a water supply on the roof, and a sink. The design was so satisfactory that another carriage was built between 1885 and 1886.

This chapter has been mainly concerned with the somewhat primitive methods of adaptation of existing railway stock for the carriage of sick and wounded troops. But we now reach the era when hospital and ambulance trains were to be specially constructed for that purpose and the next chapter deals with their earliest use by the British—in the South African War.

CHAPTER 8

Military Hospital Trains in the South African War

During the South African War of 1899–1902 trains were specially constructed for the movement of sick and wounded British troops on active service; and they were officially designated 'Hospital Trains'. It was also during this war that the British Red Cross Society began its long and valued association with the Army medical authorities in the provision, equipping and running of these trains.

When war in South Africa appeared imminent Colonel J. F. Supple, Principal Medical Officer, South Africa, initiated the conversion of ordinary trains into hospital trains. The railway system in the country was narrow gauge—3 ft 6 ins—and was practically single track throughout. One hospital train was prepared in Natal and was ready at the outbreak of war. Another was ready soon afterwards, while two more were later made up at Cape Town. Some of these trains were soon in constant use conveying casualties from Magersfontein, Modder River and Graspan to hospitals in Cape Town, De Aar and Orange River.

The hospital trains used in the first months of the war can be classified under three categories:

(a) Those which were specially fitted, equipped and staffed for the carriage of lying patients. Six were converted from ordinary rolling stock and one was specially built. These trains (generally of seven coaches each) had a staff of two medical officers, two nursing sisters, 22 other ranks, and one civilian—who was the conductor and lamp lighter.

(b) Improvised trains which were made up of first-class corridor-coaches, without alteration. These were used for the less severe cases and for convalescents, and some had a kitchen car attached. There was no permanent medical staff, but a medical officer accompanied the train when it was carrying patients.

(c) Ambulance coaches. These were specially fitted railway carriages placed at convenient intervals along the railway system. They gathered small groups of sick from various posts along the track and were then attached to passing trains and the patients offloaded at the nearest hospital. Some of these coaches had iron frames for the support of stretchers while others resembled the converted hospital train carriages.

Usually the cars were corridor-coaches, thus providing through communication. They were marshalled in the following order—one first-class saloon coach for medical officers and nursing sisters; one kitchen coach with a pharmacy and an orderlies room; three ward coaches, each of 24 beds; one ward coach with 20 beds for other ranks, and 8 screened-off beds for officers (100 patients in all); the seventh coach included a pack store and steward's store, and also had accommodation for the conductor. Water tanks, each holding about 1,800 gallons, were fitted to the staff and kitchen coaches. With the exception of the kitchen coach, all the carriages were converted Cape Government Railway bogey coaches.

The staff car had five compartments and a lavatory at each end. Two compartments were occupied by the medical officers, two by the nursing sisters, while the central compartment was used as a dining room.

The kitchen coach had three compartments, the central one being the actual kitchen fitted with a large German range and boiler. The part used as a pharmacy had four fixed wooden bunks for the staff, and the third, in addition to having bunks for six personnel, was also used as a mess room.

The ward coaches had two rows of fixed wooden bunks, each row in two tiers, and each bunk 6 ft 3 ins long and 2 ft 9 ins wide. The bottoms of the bunks were formed of tightly stretched canvas and each bunk had horsehair mattresses, blankets, pillows and sheets. All ward coaches had a lavatory, wash basin and w.c. The major portion of No 7 coach was used for the men's kit, spare blankets, linen, Red Cross stores and similar items. The steward's store was at one end and this had five bunks for personnel.

The itinerary for No 2 Hospital Train—the only one for which full details are available—shows that between 22 November, 1899, and August, 1902, it carried 10,796 patients on 226 trips. There were seven deaths on board—all of which occurred before June, 1900. The total distance covered—excluding that up country from the base—was 114,539 miles, an average of 500 miles for each journey.

Improvised hospital trains did similar work to that of the properly constructed trains except that the staff did not live on the train.

Ordinary trains were used extensively—especially for the transfer to the base of convalescent cases during the enteric fever epidemic at Bloemfontein.

Many patients in Pretoria, Johannesburg and Elandsfontein were carried by hospital train to the Natal hospitals at Newcastle, Charlestown, Howick, Pietermaritzberg and Pinetown.

25   Cots ready for loading onto the Princess Christian Hospital Train

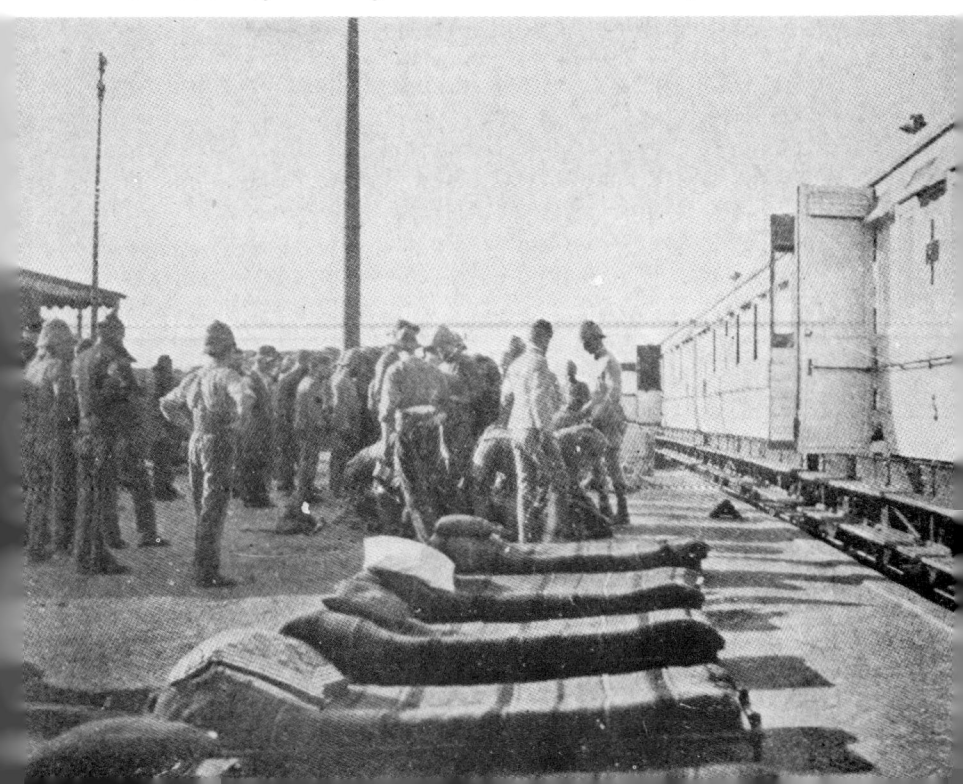

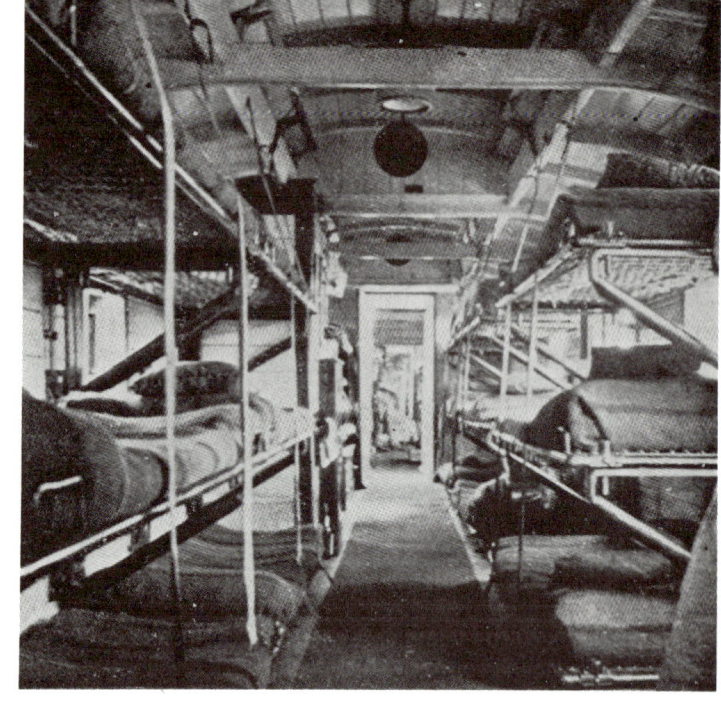

26   The interior of one of the ward cars on the Princess Christian Hospital Train

They were then transferred to Durban and embarked on hospital ships for repatriation to England.

Immediately on the outbreak of the South African War and at the suggestion of Her Royal Highness Princess Christian of Schleswig-Holstein, the Central Red Cross Committee on Voluntary Organization voted money towards building and equipping a complete hospital train. Additional money was collected by Princess Christian, who herself made a donation; other contributors included the Royal Borough of Windsor, the Worcester Red Cross Committee and the people of Canada.

The train was constructed by the Birmingham Carriage and Wagon Company, the contract being signed on 18 October, 1899. Sir John Furley,* who had made a study of the transport of the sick and wounded and had seen Prussian hospital trains in use in the Franco–Prussian War, was responsible for the general design and internal arrangements. W. J. Fieldhouse, the managing director of the Military Equipment Company, took responsibility for its actual construction. The train was the first hospital train to be built in England and, at the request of the

* Furley, with Lechmere and Duncan, founded the Ambulance Department of the Order of St John of Jerusalem in 1888.

Royal Borough of Windsor, it was named the 'Princess Christian Hospital Train'. Its construction details are given in Appendix G.

The train was commanded by Surgeon Lieutenant-Colonel F. S. Forrestor, with Mr P. Lowe FRCS as second medical officer, and two nursing sisters, while the orderlies were members of the St John Ambulance Brigade.

Its first trip was to Ladysmith and was made on the night of 18 March, 1900. It was planned that it should inaugurate the opening of the trestle bridge which had been temporarily placed over the Tugela River at Colenso. It did so, but had to wait for half an hour while the last bolt was driven into the bridge. It was the first train to reach Ladysmith since the siege, and on the following morning entrained its first load of patients—ten officers from Ladysmith and 54 other ranks from a camp at Intombi. The patients were taken to Durban, where they were transferred to the Hospital Ship *German*.

Throughout its period of service in South Africa, which was mainly on the Natal side of the Pretoria line, the hospital train carried over 7,500 patients. There were altogether six deaths on the train—three patients and three of the staff—during the 108 journeys which totalled 42,000 miles.

27 One of the 'Netley Coaches'; the author served on these coaches from 1914–16

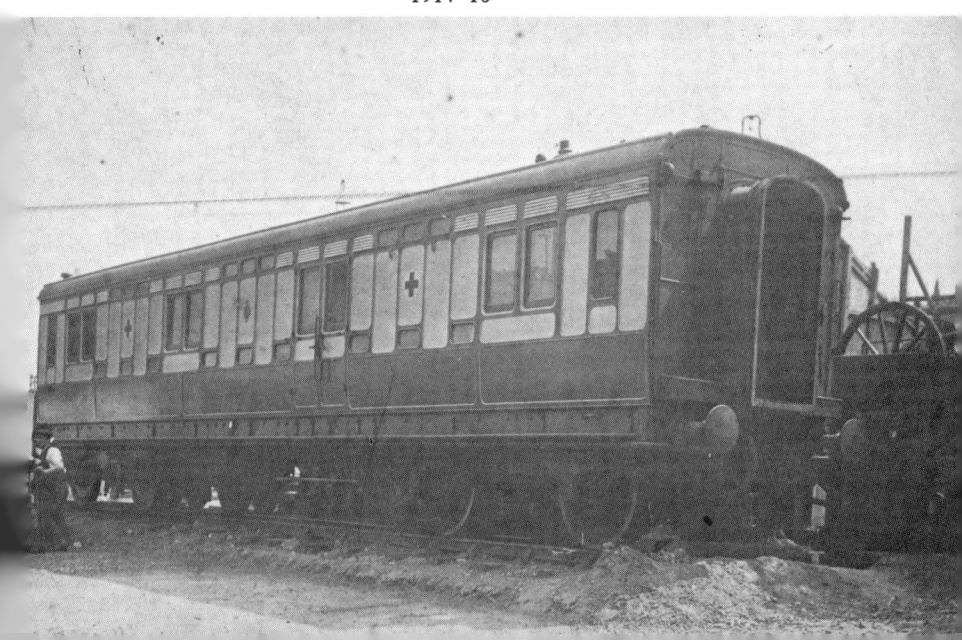

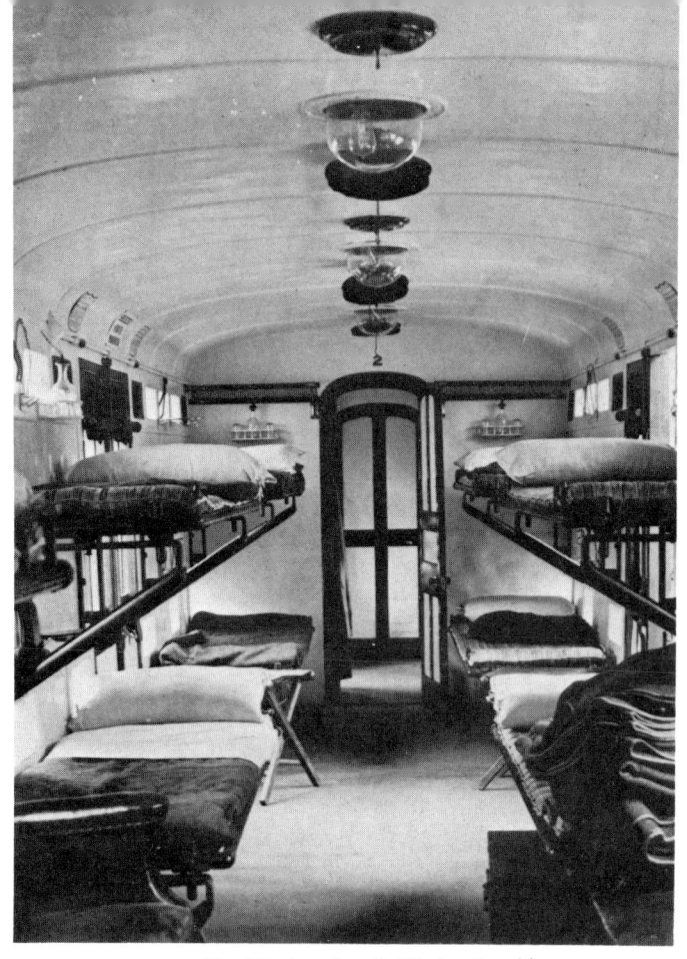

28   The interior of a 'Netley Coach'

In June, 1901, the 'Princess Christian Hospital Train' was presented by the Central Red Cross Committee to the Secretary of State for War on the understanding that it should retain its name 'Princess Christian Hospital Train' and remain as a complete unit for the military forces in South Africa. Eventually two of its coaches formed the nucleus of an ambulance train in South-West Africa in the First World War.

In April, 1900, the Principal Medical Officer of the Field Force, Surgeon-General Sir W. D. Wilson, asked Sir John Furley (who was then Chief Commissioner of the British Red Cross Society) to supply another hospital train. Under his supervision and with the assistance of Dr E. Stewart a somewhat improvised train was made up at East London. It became No 4 Hospital Train, and its details are given in Appendix H.

No 4 Hospital Train came into service on 10 June, 1900, carrying 78 patients from East London to Bloemfontein. Altogether it travelled more than 114,000 miles and carried nearly 11,000 patients, commanded by Dr Stewart and assisted by two sisters and 12 orderlies.

The Boers also used four complete hospital trains during the South African War. They adapted these from the rolling stock in the central workshops of the Netherlands South African Railway at Pretoria.

In 1900 five railway 'ambulance coaches' were designed by Major W. D. Macpherson RAMC (later Major-General Sir William) and constructed in England by the London and South Western Railway Company. They were garaged at the railway siding of the Royal Victoria Hospital, Netley, and known officially as the 'War Department Ambulance Train'—but more affectionately by the troops as the 'Netley Coaches'. Their first use was to carry casualties from the South African War who arrived at Southampton to Netley and other hospitals in England. Their description is given in Appendix P.

Before ending the pre-First World War era, mention should be made of the 8th International Conference of Red Cross Societies which was held at the Princess Hall in Earl's Court in June, 1907. There were about 200 exhibits concerned with the transport of wounded, and these naturally included railway ambulance transport vehicles. The largest contribution at the Exhibition came from the German Red Cross Society.

CHAPTER 9

Military Ambulance Trains on Service Overseas in the First World War

When mobilization plans were being prepared before the outbreak of the First World War the Army Medical Department made provision for the construction and supply of ambulance trains—not only for the theatre of war but also for use at home. In the 'Organization of an Expeditionary Force of Six Divisions for Overseas—1907' six ambulance trains were included, their lay-out and construction having been decided in committee well before there was a threatened outbreak of hostilities. In the South African War these units had been called 'Hospital Trains'; the name 'Ambulance Train' was used in the First World War and thereafter.

Their general role was to collect the sick and wounded from the front and take them to base hospitals or to ports for embarkation in hospital ships. Occasionally the front would be a railhead just behind the firing line but generally the patients were to be collected from Casualty Clearing Stations well behind the actual front line.

No properly constructed ambulance trains were immediately ready for shipment overseas when war was declared and it was therefore intended that the transport of British casualties from the fighting areas to the French ports would be made in French *trains sanitaires*. The trains were to be prepared in France and each would consist of 33 special goods trucks *(fourgons de marchandise)* with brake vans for stores, office and dispensary, a restaurant car or van fitted up as a kitchen, and first and second class coaches for personnel. Each truck was to be fitted with four frames of the 'Bréchot-Déspres-Amelines' stretcher-carrying apparatus—thus providing each train with accom-

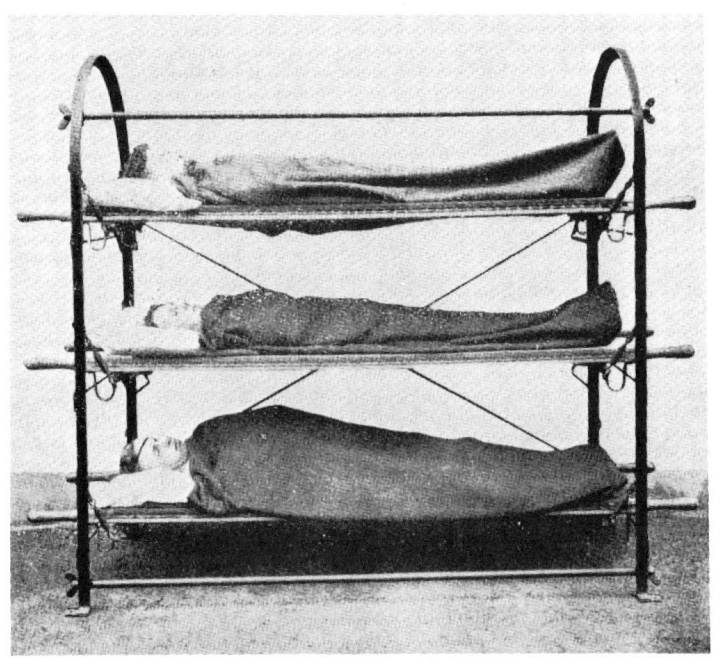

29 The Bréchot–Déspres–Amelines stretcher-carrying apparatus with three lying-down patients

modation for 396 'cot' patients. A number of sets of this apparatus had been despatched to France from the United Kingdom with the earliest supply ships and they could be installed in practically any type of railway vehicle. Briefly, the apparatus was made of iron and consisted of two very strong but light uprights, each bent into the shape of an inverted and elongated 'U'. The uprights were placed six feet from each other and were connected by horizontal rods or stays; each leg had an expanded foot which was bolted to the floor of the carriage. Each frame could carry three patients on stretchers in tiers, and when the frames were not in use they could be folded and up to 40 sets carried in an empty truck. See illustrations 29 and 30.

However, because of their own heavy casualties, high losses of rolling stock to the advancing Germans and the shortage of

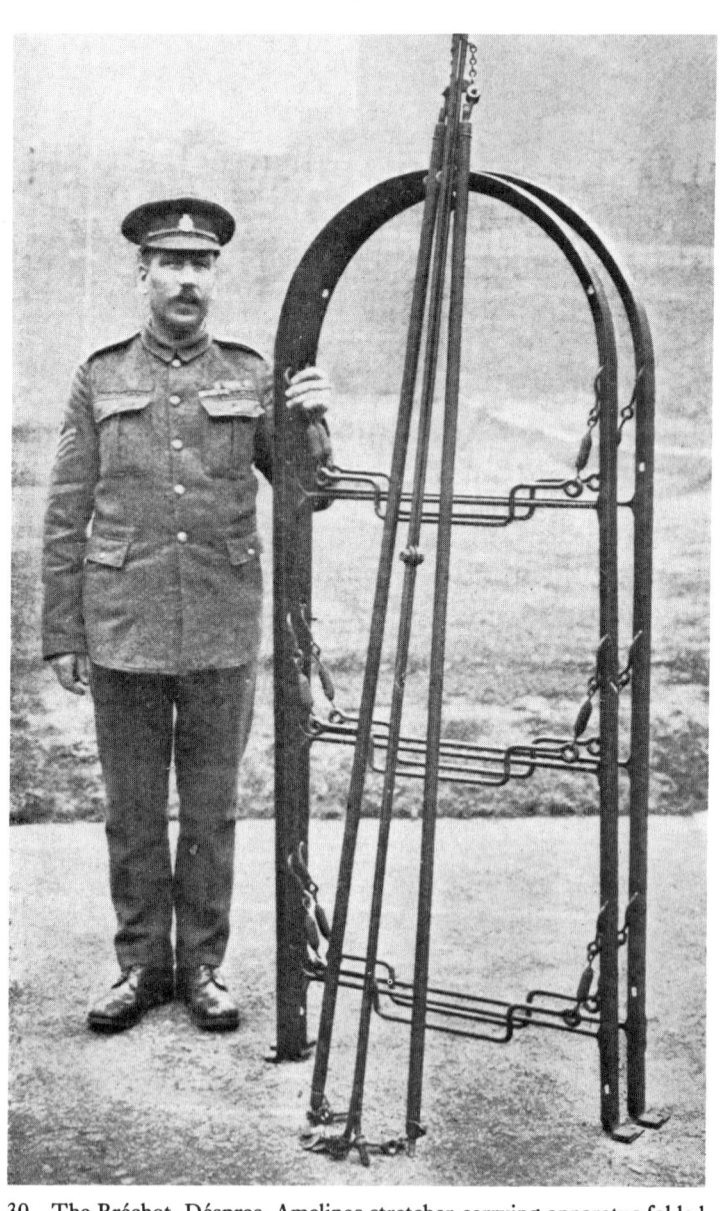

30 The Bréchot–Déspres–Amelines stretcher-carrying apparatus folded for transport

their own railway staff, the French had no *'trains sanitaires'* to spare for British troops. So adaptation and improvisation became essential, ambulance trains being made up of any available carriages, coaches, vans, covered trucks or other rolling stock from the French railways in which the 'Bréchot-Déspres-Amelines' apparatus could be installed.

Before any of these could be brought into use, casualties were evacuated—as in earlier wars—in cattle trucks; sometimes they lay on straw, at other times on mattresses, and occasionally there was the luxury of convent pillows.

How did these improvised ambulance trains actually come into being? In August, 1914, six detachments of RAMC ambulance train personnel (totalling about 300) had joined at Aldershot where they were trained in their duties, collected medical stores and other equipment, and then crossed to France. They reached Amiens on 15 August, 1914, and by the 17th, at a large railway junction about one mile distant, 100 goods wagons and a few passenger carriages were handed over by the French. These formed the beginning of the British ambulance train service with the BEF.

The train crews immediately got to work dividing the rolling stock into three trains. Carriages were cleaned and disinfected and four sets of Bréchot-Déspres-Amelines apparatus fixed in each empty wagon, each therefore providing accommodation for 12 lying cases. The design of the apparatus, incidentally, counteracted to a remarkable degree the jolting of these heavy wagons.

Within a few days each train had clean, well-equipped wards, dispensaries and surgical dressing rooms, as well as accommodation for stores and equipment, food, reserve stretchers and blankets. Ovens and stoves capable of cooking for over 700 patients were installed in converted restaurant cars, the iron chimneys leading out of the roofs. Barrels for fresh water, disinfecting apparatus, filters and ice-chests were also installed. And so Nos 1, 2 and 3 British Ambulance Trains were born—not completely equipped, but well able to do their job. As all the necessary medical supplies, blankets, reserve stretchers, pails, jugs, basins, camp stoves, etc, were not immediately available from British Ordnance Depots—resort was made to 'local purchase'. This involved three train commanders going on a foray and scouring the shops in Amiens, while another train commander went to Paris for items not available in Amiens.

While these trains were being completed, medical aid was supplied on the food trains which travelled daily to and from the front. Twelve folded sets of Bréchot-Déspres-Amelines apparatus, with medical and surgical panniers and other appliances, were put in one of the vans in each supply train going to the front, under the charge of an NCO and three RAMC orderlies. Before the return journey the vans were scrubbed and disinfected, the apparatus erected, and provision thus made for 36 lying and about 80 sitting cases to be evacuated to the rear.

Eventually Nos 1, 2 and 3 trains were completed and made their first journeys to the front on 24, 25 and 26 August respectively. Work on a fourth train was immediately put in hand, this being made up of third class carriages from which the seats had been removed. The moment it was ready it was sent to Rouen and came into service on 30 August.

Railway carriages, vans, trucks, wagons—in fact any form of railway stock—meant everything to the medical personnel, and they were obtained by whatever means possible. So the principal task at this period was asking anyone in authority for railway vehicles to make additional trains. These efforts achieved little, so that the next approach was to the French Government for the loan of one of their temporary ambulance trains. But this was during the retreat from Mons and there was, therefore, extreme pressure on the whole French army. Their requirements were as great as, if not greater than, Britain's, and sanction for a train could not be obtained.

However, a compromise soon presented itself, for a French ambulance train arrived on the scene and the urgent needs of our ambulance train transport for the British troops was explained to the Commandant. The result was that 45 RAMC personnel, together with four truckloads of stores and equipment, were merged with the French train which had its own staff of officers and 25 men. On 31 August this composite *'Entente Cordiale'* train moved to the fighting area around

Paris. On arrival at Creil—which had also been reached by Nos 2, 3 and 4 British trains—there was a share-out of equipment. The *'Entente Cordiale'* was then re-designated the 'Franco-British' and it made its first journey to Verneuil l'Etang on 5 September. Here it entrained the sick and wounded from three field ambulances, as well as some prisoners-of-war and a group of captured spies. It then headed for the port of St Nazaire and was to take 64 hours for the journey. First, though, on 8 September the train reached Coulommiers, where it took on 80 seriously wounded patients who had been brought to the railhead in horsedrawn supply wagons of the Army Service Corps.

By this time the 'Franco-British' had virtually become a hospital on wheels. Groups of carriages had been portioned off as surgical and medical wards. Store rooms and offices were installed and the well-equipped kitchens were in full swing. Close harmony between the French and British train crews ensured that the train was a success.

Unfortunately there was no system of inter-communication between the carriages, though this was overcome by the orderlies moving along the side footboards outside the carriages, often while the train was in motion.

On arrival at St Nazaire on 10 September the patients were transferred to the ill-fated Hospital Ship *Asturias*. Shortly afterwards, for the sake of convenience, the 'Franco-British' was again redesignated—this time it became No 6 Ambulance Train.

The need for additional ambulance trains became greater than ever and two trains were promised to be at Le Mans on 13 September. There was another scouring of the local shops for supplies, which then had to be taken to Villeneuve as the trains had moved there from Le Mans. Further purchases were made in Villeneuve and on 15 September No 5 Ambulance Train left for the front, completely equipped and fully staffed. Two days later No 7 Ambulance Train was also on its way to the forward area. This was one of the first ambulance trains to be involved in enemy action. One the night of 1–2 November, at the height of the Battle of Ypres, it was under bombardment with high explosive and shrapnel while entraining seriously wounded patients at Ypres railway station. The train suffered severe damage, with wrecked coachwork and broken windows, and it was unable to move to safety because the engine had been taken down the line to Hazebrouck in search of water. The bombardment was not, however, permitted to interfere with the attendance to the wounded on the train and the application of dressings and other treatment continued in the normal way.

There was now heavy fighting in progress on the River Aisne as well and 1,500 patients were evacuated through Villeneuve on 18 September. In those early days of the war casualties often came to the Ambulance Trains direct from the fighting line, covered in mud and with only a first field dressing on their wounds.

Early on 21 September, a Red Cross ambulance train, composed of *wagons-lit* and a restaurant car (all representative of the best French rolling stock) arrived. Another similar train appeared two hours later. As the accommodation on each was only 200 cases—far too few for the immediate requirements on the one very thronged line to the front—the trains were joined together. 30 orderlies were added to the staff and the train made one journey in this capacity. Afterwards all the vehicles were merged into those of other trains, this being considered to give better utilization.

As the conflict progressed, British ambulance trains became much more efficient and comfortable; nursing sisters were regularly doing duty on them and there were ample supplies of stores and comforts of all kinds. With winter approaching, however, the question of light and warmth became urgent, so lighting and heating equipment was obtained from the Flamme Bleu Company in Paris. Stoves were placed in corridors and wards, the surrounding woodwork being protected by iron or asbestos.

Meanwhile carriages and other vehicles were still being collected at Villeneuve and on 8 October No 8 Ambulance Train made its first trip. Three more large restaurant cars were obtained from the French railway authorities and each was adapted to accommodate 18 to 24 badly wounded cases. These cars were loaded through their broad side-windows—the plate glass having been substituted with light wooden shutters.

On 12 October several large luggage vans were obtained from the P.L.M. Railway Company and these were soon converted into well-heated and comfortable ward cars and kitchens. When additional vans became available the familiar routine of cleaning, disinfecting, painting and fitting 'BDA' stretcher-bearing apparatus followed. No 9 train made its first trip on 31 October and No 10 on 13 November.

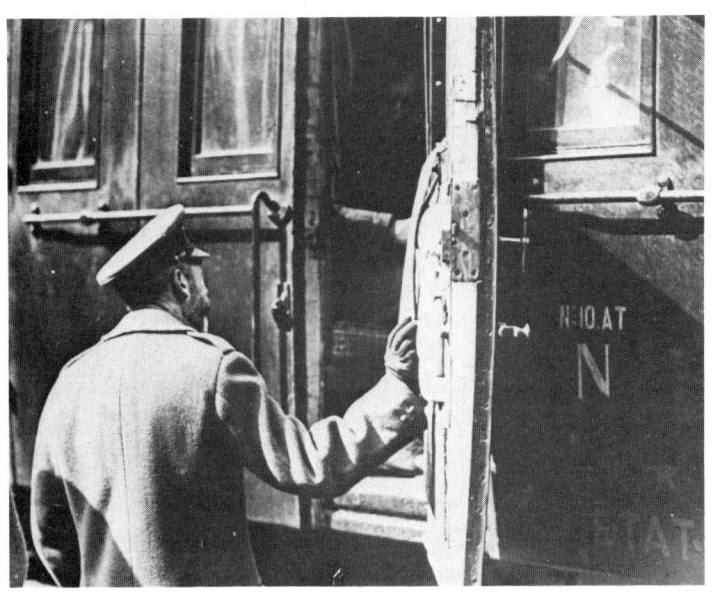

31 King George V talking to patients in No 10 British Ambulance Train, one of the early BEF ambulance trains that was constructed from French 'Etat' rolling stock. It could carry 280 lying-down patients and 180 sitting cases

Casualties were so great, however, that many were arriving from the front in empty supply trains, frequently still with only a covering of straw on the floor. Many of the trucks were of the '8 Chevaux—40 Hommes' variety so well known by our troops in France. These trucks had carried the horses of the BEF to the forward areas and there were many thousands of them with the early divisions. Since the horses needed straw, there was an adequate supply for the wounded troops.

At this time the British Red Cross Committee requested the assistance of Sir John Furley, then 78 years of age, and W. J. Fieldhouse (who had been responsible for the construction of hospital trains in the South African War) in producing an ambulance train in France. An Engineering draughtsman accompanied Sir John to Rouen, where drawings were made for the conversion of 15 third-class coaches of French rolling stock into a train. The plans and drawings were sent to the Birmingham Carriage and Railway Wagon Company, where fittings were made under the supervision of Mr Fieldhouse; these were then sent back to Rouen where the train was completed. This improvised train was not entirely satisfactory because once again there were no connecting passages between the coaches. Each coach had to be treated as an almost self-supporting ward, with its own staff and equipment. When possible, more serious cases were kept together, the staff being supplemented from the personnel in other coaches at the frequent stopping places. The British Red Cross Society contributed nearly £4,000 towards the cost of this train which started service on 15 December, 1914, as No 11—and was the last to be made up from rolling stock. It remained in service for four years and on one occasion was ahead of the British artillery and just behind the line of machine guns, while an imminent German advance was awaited.

In mid-December the Commanding Officers of all the improvised ambulance trains—who for months had lived on and administered them—gave their views as to what improvements they considered necessary. All the heavy vehicles of Nos 1, 2 and 3 were replaced by first and second class carriages from the various French railway systems. These carriages were used for the more seriously wounded cases—some of whose stretchers were comfortably suspended on springs—while others were able to lie down on the seats, which had been broadened. Third class carriages accommodated the sitting cases while skin, infectious, mental and other special cases were segregated in separate compartments. At this time each train carried up to 800 patients and had a complete staff of officers, nurses and orderlies. There were two kitchens on each train, one near one end and the other in the middle.

Before dealing with the arrival in France of properly constructed ambulance trains from the United Kingdom and the use of railway ambulance transport in other theatres of war, two stories graphically illustrate conditions at that time.

The first, although not actually about the running of ambulance trains, certainly concerns what happened to one train load of patients. It was told by Major G. A. Moore RAMC, who was Officer Commanding Ambulance Trains in France at the time. Under the pseudonym 'Wagon-Lit' he wrote, in 1916, an article entitled 'The Birth and early days of our ambulance trains in France—August, 1914' which appeared in the 1921 issue of the *Journal of the Royal Army Medical Corps*.

'At the large railway station at Villeneuve Triage' Wagon-Lit wrote, 'we had no hospital but only a slightly equipped medical aid post for the treatment of the local sick. Heavy fighting was now in progress on the River Aisne and ambulance trains full of wounded kept continually passing through our station; 1,500 cases on September 18 alone. On the 17th one such stopped with imperative orders to us to unload it and return it at once to the front. The situation for us on that day was not a simple one. Over 150 stretcher cases alone required carrying by hand to our aid post, a distance of over half a mile in pelting rain. To transfer and attend to these patients we had only 3 medical officers, 6 orderlies and 2 cooks. Things looked black indeed when "out of the blue" appeared 250 of the London Scottish who had just arrived, heard of our difficulties and offered their services. All through the day and night these splendid men worked for us and by 7 pm we had been able to get the worst of 150 cases under shelter and fed, and had begun to dress their wounds. Little headway could the three medical officers and six orderlies have made among such numbers had not again the marvellous happened. Up to the door of our aid post came an officer in Red Cross uniform. He explained that he was Dr Braithwaite in charge of the American ambulance at Neuilly: that hearing of our difficulty he had motored from Paris with three other surgeons, instruments, ample dressings, etc., and that he wished to place himself at our service in every way, and finally that he had ordered his fleet of motor ambulances (the first I had seen in France) to follow him out to us. In these he promised to take to Paris hospitals any of our cases requiring operation. I gratefully accepted his offer and the removal of the most suitable cases commenced at once.

As if by magic, out of the ranks of the London Scottish stepped four sergeants and privates, all qualified doctors, also some medical students and with them their regimental surgeon, the gallant Captain McNab who was killed in action a little later on while attending to one of his beloved "London Scotties" in their front trenches. From somewhere too, I know not where, dropped three qualified lady doctors—fine they were, and splendidly they worked all night and day, snatching a few hours sleep in a truck. What a transformation! Our large aid post shed which up to 11.30 that morning had been occupied by some half dozen light cases, at 4.30 pm was a huge and well-lighted ward with some 200 patients (officers and men), many of whom were dangerously wounded. Looking after them you would have seen 12 surgeons, male and female, 6 Royal Army Medical Corps orderlies and 100 volunteers from the London Scottish. From time to time motor ambulances kept arriving to take the cases to Paris, and by nightfall ninety of the worst were in bed and comfort at Neuilly. Long before dawn the remainder had been dressed and given their much needed sleep. In my recollection this day will always stand out as "Miracle Day" '.

The second story is taken from the *Diary of a Nursing Sister on the Western Front—1914/1915* and was written by Sister K. E. Luard RRC, who served in France throughout the war, and it deals with the running of one of the earliest trains during the first days of the war until late March, 1915.

In those early days when it was said that an ambulance train went up to the front it meant exactly that. Improvised ambulance trains went up the railway line as far as it would take them, often within the vicinity of the front, and occasionally bringing them under enemy attack.

Sister Luard was posted to an improvised ambulance train

on 13 October, 1914; her immediate impression was that it appeared to be about a third of a mile in length, had lovely ward beds and pillows, pillow cases and blankets, and adequate supplies of medical and other equipment. Her colleagues on the train were three medical officers, three other nursing sisters and three RAMC orderlies to each ward coach. The train seems to have been employed non-stop from the time she joined it at Braisne until the end of March, 1915. She lists the entraining stations as Amiens, Bailleul, Béthune, Blendeque, Chocques, Hazebrouck, La Bassée, Lillers, Merville, Nieppe, Poperinghe, St Omer and Steenwerck. The patients were carried to Boulogne, Le Havre or Rouen for embarkation on hospital ships, or to Etaples, Etretat, Le Mans, Marseilles, Paris, Villeneuve, Versailles and elsewhere for admission to general and other hospitals.

On one occasion during the early days of the war, three trains made up of cattle trucks carried 1,175 wounded (510 in one train) from the front. The patients were lying on straw and had been in the train for several days. Only once had their wounds been dressed. On arrival at the railway station fresh dressings were applied and the patients sorted into categories—either for admission to local medical units or for evacuation to the base. One of the trains going to the base at St Nazaire had 141 patients on board under the charge of a medical officer, Sister Luard, another nursing sister and two RAMC orderlies. The most serious cases were put in the trucks next to the nursing sisters, who could only attend to them when the train stopped at a station or elsewhere; and only at the station stops was it possible to give the patients some sort of a meal. This story is exceptional because at this time there were at least five improvised ambulance trains in service but all were on other sectors of the front.

Obviously in those early days the vast majority of all patients had been wounded in combat and many were dangerously ill. Many of the fractured femur cases reached the train in riflesplints—the traditional emergency method of splinting such cases, *vide* the instructions in the RAMC Training Manual of 1911. Fractured femurs were one of the hazards suffered by the numerous mounted troops.

Even as late as 14 January, 1915, Sister Luard recalled, the badly wounded who were loaded on the trains at Béthune were caked in mud up to their necks, and two months later a train filled up at the front with wounded men who were practically asleep on their feet from exhaustion.

Not all the patients were battle casualties. Already many were suffering from frost-bite, influenza, pneumonia, rheumatism or trench feet. Others had contracted diphtheria, enteric fever, malaria, measles, mumps or scarlet fever—thus showing the necessity of having separate accommodation for infectious patients. There were many Indian troops on this sector of the front and an additional problem was segregating those of different castes. Sometimes French civilian and women casualties were entrained; once there was a French girl of 16 who had lost an arm, and a woman of 61 minus a foot.

As was to be expected, Sister Luard's train had many teething troubles. Very early on there was a shortage of water, and at the same time the gas supply ran out, leaving candles as the only illuminant. Later the train had to be divided into three sections to facilitate the unloading of patients. On one almost comical occasion early in December, two railway engines were attached to the train—one at each end—and when they tried to move off in opposite directions there was an obvious stalemate. Then they both reversed—with the unfortunate result that three coaches were put out of action. Later, on account of bad shunting, the kitchen car became detached and the train had to make one journey without it. In mid-November, however, the heating, gas and water supplies of the train were overhauled at Sotteville and electric lighting was installed.

Even during the infrequent occasions when the train was standing by awaiting its next journey, there was plenty for the staff to do. On 26 November a French railway engine arrived with a red cross on it, so a few days later Sister Luard and other members of the staff began painting red crosses on the sides of the train.

It is apparent from the diary that the writer could speak French, and as early as 22 August she records talking with local inhabitants. Later, in February, 1915, she instituted French classes among the staff of the train—17 members attended lessons in the men's mess-coach and made good progress. To help dealing with her Indian patients Sister Luard started to learn Hindustani!

Sister Luard's diary is a heart-rending tribute to the suffering and bravery of the wounded troops and clearly shows their incredible cheerfulness.

At the end of March, 1915, Sister Luard was posted to a field ambulance, a most unusual posting for a nursing sister. She appears to have remained with it only until May, 1915, and then, after four months at a base hospital, she was sent up the line to a casualty clearing station on 17 October, 1915, as Sister-in-Charge.

Her second book, *Unknown Warriors,* covers the period from this date until 11 August, 1918, and in it she is continually referring to the evacuation of patients from her casualty clearing station to ambulance trains. Here is one extract:

'Palm Sunday. 24 March, 1918 (at the time of the German Advance). At about 5 pm the Railway Transport Officer of the ruined village produced a train with 50 trucks of the "8 Chevaux—40 Hommes" pattern and ran it alongside the camp. Not enough of course for the wounded of both hospitals but enough to make some impression. Never was a dirty old empty truck train given a more eager welcome or greeted with more profound relief. The 150 walking cases (all the rest were stretcher patients) were got into open trucks and the stretchers quickly loaded into others with an orderly, a pail of water, feeders and other necessaries ... I got a supply of morphine and hypodermics to use at the stoppages all down the train ... The medical officers took the morphia ... There were 300 stretcher cases left but another train was coming in for them. Thus even at the end of the war improvisation of the most elementary kind was necessary in the evacuation of wounded by railway transport.'

We can now continue with the arrival of properly constructed ambulance trains from the United Kingdom. No 12 was the first and arrived on 12 November, 1914. It had been

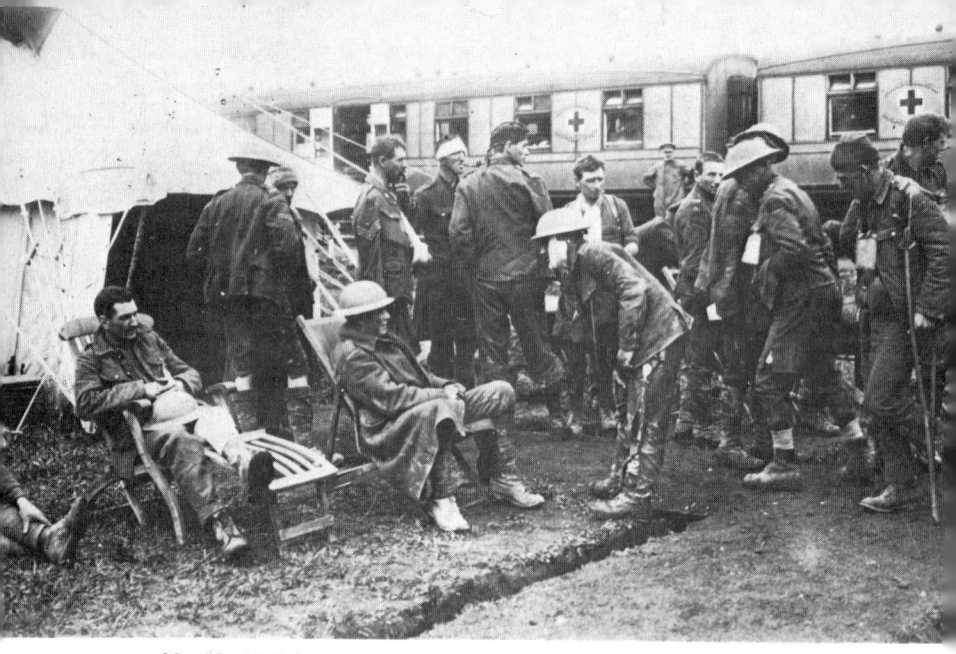

32 No 15 Princess Christian Hospital Train which entered service on 1 June, 1915. This illustration shows the evacuation of Canadian wounded on the Western Front in 1916

made up of vehicles of some of the home ambulance trains and because of its outside colour was known as the 'Khaki' train. No train was numbered 13 so No 14 was the next to arrive. It was given by Lord and Lady Michelham, called 'Queen Mary's Ambulance Train' and was soon followed by Nos 15 to 18, 21, 22 and 24.

No 15 train cost £25,000 and this was defrayed by Princess Christian; like its predecessor in the South African War it was then designated the 'Princess Christian Hospital Train'. It was made up of ten coaches, to which the War Office added two more for sitting patients. Like the train sent to South Africa it was constructed by the Birmingham Carriage and Railway Wagon Company, again under the personal direction of Sir John Furley, and once more with the practical assistance of W. J. Fieldhouse. Unlike the other ambulance trains, which were adapted from normal rolling stock, the 'Princess Christian Hospital Train' was specially constructed for its purpose. It had one other distinction—the other trains were 'ambulance' trains, but this was a 'hospital' train, and this was painted on each side of all the coaches.

The arrangement of the wards followed the design of the earlier South African train. They contained Furley-Fieldhouse cots which were supported on brackets in tiers and were capable of being removed to be used as stretchers. The cots could also be turned back to make a comfortable seat, and each bed had a bracket for a cup and a glass. The wards—each accommodating 36 patients—had moveable wash-basins. A main kitchen, subsidiary kitchen, surgery, and a mess and sleeping accommodation for the staff were also included. The train had gas and electric lighting, and was steam heated from the engine. Its total length was 700 feet.

This train was unique in the fact that a mechanic was engaged from the Great Western Railway Company to accompany it to France to do running repairs. Three men who were trained in restaurant-car duties were added to the staff of the train. These orderlies continued to draw pay from the Princess Christian fund until near the end of 1918, when the British Red Cross Joint War Committee took over the responsibility.

The United Kingdom Flour Millers Association provided ambulance trains Nos 16 and 17, which were specially built and equipped at a cost of about £24,000. They were constructed under the direction of the Railway Executive Committee from plans approved by the War Office and embodied the latest developments in railway ambulance transport.

The expenses of running Nos 11, 16 and 17 were borne jointly by the Army, the Friends Ambulance Unit and the Joint Committee of the British Red Cross Society and the Order of St John. The charge to the Joint War Committee was in respect of wages, subsistence, repairs, renewals and stores. With the exception of the Commanding Officer, who was a medical officer of the RAMC, these three trains were staffed entirely by British Red Cross personnel and Friends Ambulance orderlies. These men replaced the BRCS orderlies who enlisted into the RAMC at the end of 1915.

A further ten ambulance trains—Nos 19 and 20, 23, and 25 to 31, reached France in 1916. Eight more, Nos 32 to 38 and No 41 arrived in 1917, while the last three trains to go to France, Nos 9, 42 and 43, reached their destination in the last year of the war.

The thirteen ambulance trains numbered 26 to 38 were of a standard pattern produced in 1916, and were constructed on

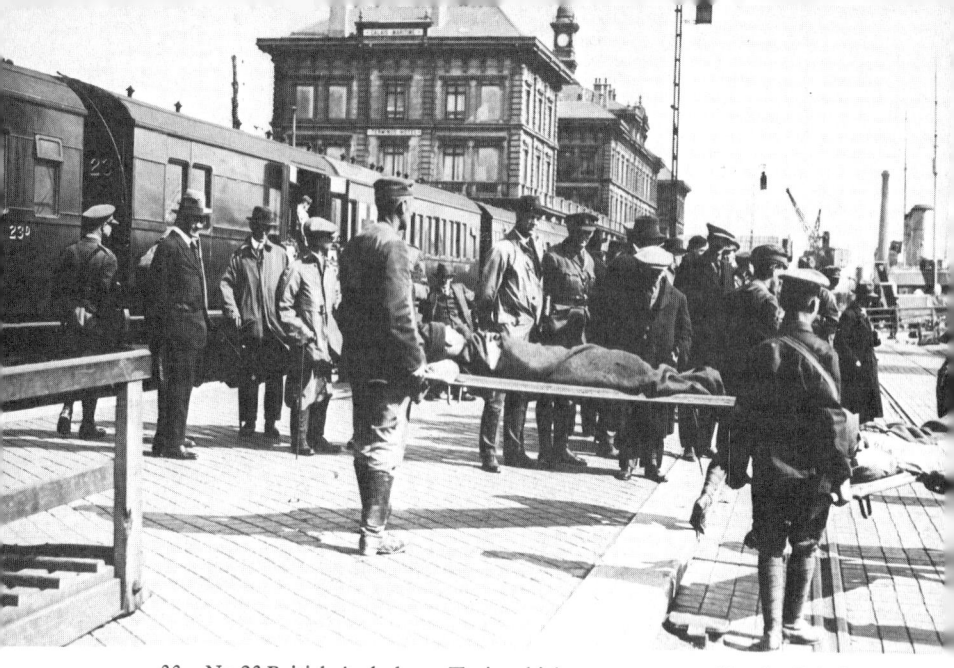

33   No 23 British Ambulance Train which was constructed by the Caledonian Railway Company and entered service in France on 3 March, 1916. This picture shows patients being detrained at Calais on 2 September, 1918 for transfer to a hospital ship and embarkation for England

34   No 39 British Ambulance Train: walking wounded being entrained at Hinges on 10 April, 1918 during a German offensive. This train, one of the standard ambulance trains, was sent to France at the end of 1917. It was made up of sixteen coaches and could carry 356 stretcher cases and some 'sitters'.
  The author served on this train in France and Italy from 1917 to 1919

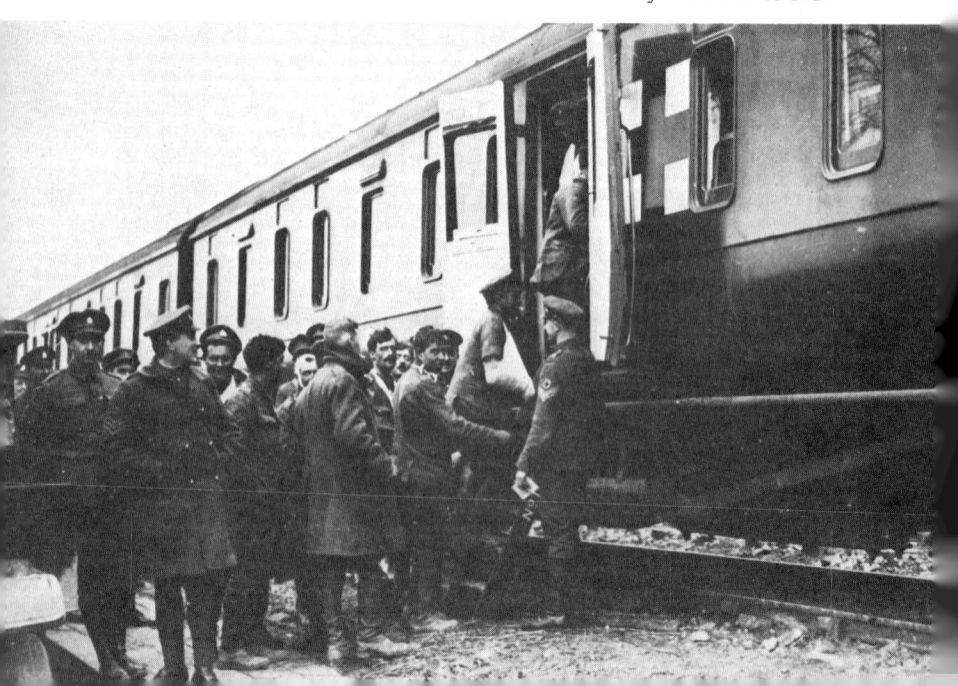

the recommendations of an Ambulance Train Committee which had been set up in France to consider the views of the medical officers who had commanded ambulance trains from the very early days of the war. Four other trains, Nos 39, 41, 42 and 43, were constructed to the same general standard—but with increased accommodation for stretcher patients.

The description in Appendix M applies in general to all these standard ambulance trains.

An Ambulance Train Depot and Supply Store was established at Abbeville on 1 April, 1917. It was responsible for all British ambulance trains in France, and provided them with stores and medical and other equipment. It also dealt with train personnel questions and liaised with the French railway

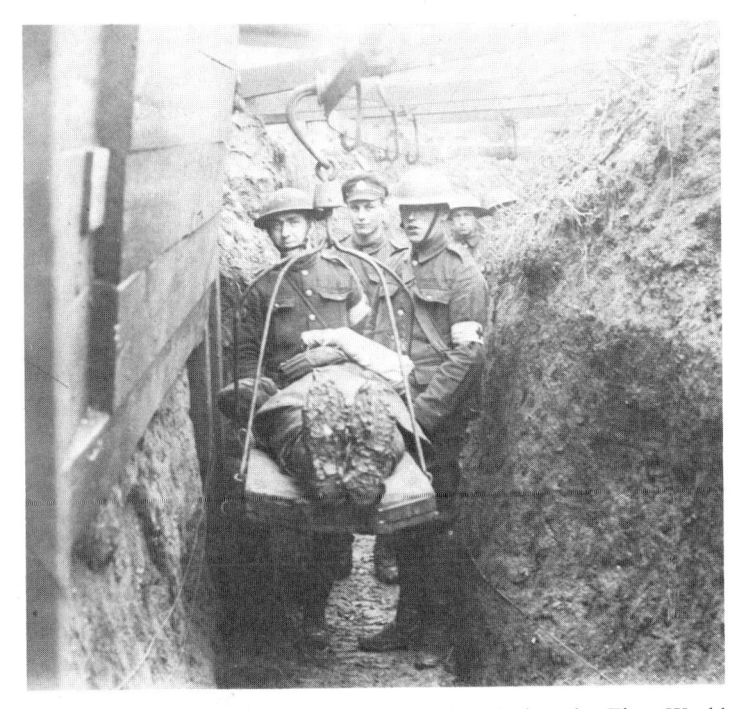

35 Carriage of the wounded in the trenches during the First World War—one of the methods by which British casualties were carried from the battle area was by means of an overhead trolley

authorities for repairs to the rolling stock. Prior to this a *fourgon,* which contained a reserve of medical and surgical supplies, stretchers and blankets, had been attached to each train.

In June, 1916, temporary ambulance trains, numbered 100 upwards, were taken into service in France. They were made up of twenty-one first, second and third class coaches, and each accommodated 1,000 patients, mostly sitting cases.

Other types of rail ambulance included 'trench railways' which were first constructed in France in 1915—being used at Festubert in May that year and at Loos in the following September. A divisional trench tramway officer was responsible not only for maintaining the tramway line but also for supplying mules! Monorails were also used to carry the wounded along deep trenches.

Small special ambulance trains were used on the 'Decauville' system, each consisting of an engine, two covered hospital trucks which each accommodated 12 lying patients, and an open truck for 24 sitters, a total of 48 patients in each train.

Other improvised ambulance trains on narrow gauge systems on the Frévant-Avèsnes line comprised an engine and six carriages or eight trucks, each train being able to accommodate 108 patients.

The Canadian Army Medical Service had their own system of 'tram-cars' for the cariage of patients along a sunken road from an advanced dressing station. These 'tram-cars' accommodated 40 casualties and were drawn by mules—which were normally sheltered in dug-outs off the sunken road.

During 1917 and 1918 covered bogie wagons were built for use on the rear section of the forward light railways and for the Trouville hospital railway. They were bascially intended for ambulance use, each carrying eight stretcher cases and four walking wounded. But the ambulance fittings could easily be removed, allowing the wagons to revert to ordinary use. Each of the vans actually carried nine stretchers—two tiers of three along the sides at one end of the vehicle and one tier of three at the other end, facing a single longitudinal folding seat. One of the stretchers, however, was used solely for the carriage of kits. There was sufficient room in each wagon for the orderlies to

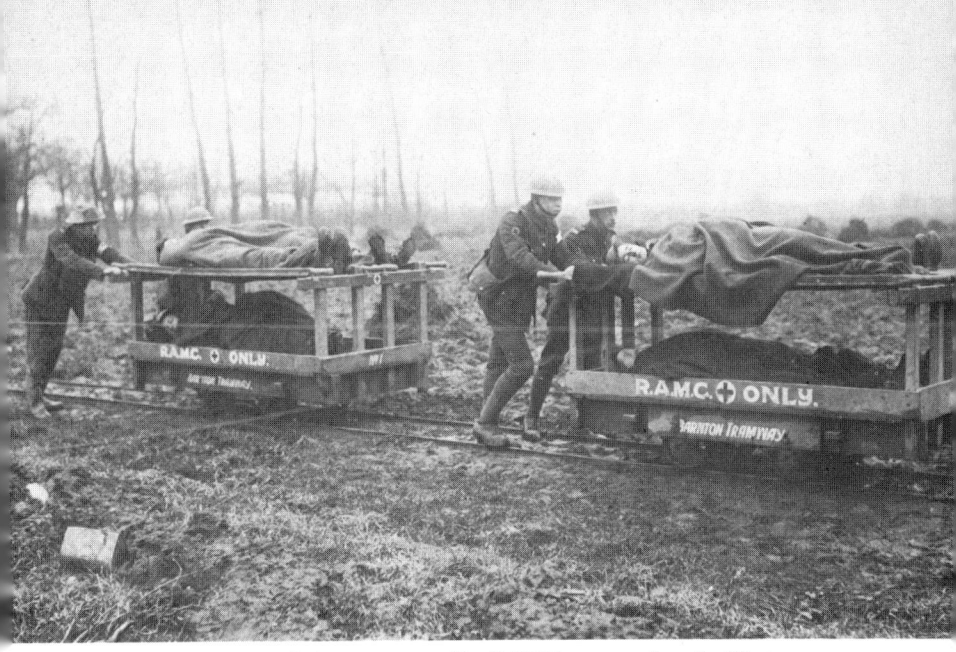

36 Stretcher cases being transported by RAMC personnel on the Western Front by means of a Barnton Tramway on a narrow gauge railway track

tend the patients and the stretcher brackets and seats were made to fold up against the sides of the wagons. There were narrow sliding doors at each end to enable the staff to move from one vehicle to another when the train was moving.

Before dealing with the use of ambulance trains in other theatres of war, the following figures give some indication of the magnitude of the task of ambulance trains in France in the early days of the war. It deals only with the evacuation of casualties from the forward areas to the rear:

From 14 to 29 September, 1914, nearly 8,250 patients were evacuated from the Aisne, the majority in the six improvised ambulance trains available, but some in troop trains.

In the same year, from 15 October to 23 November, when 11 improvised trains were available, 138,000 casualties were brought down from the Flanders front.

The Battle of Neuve Chapelle resulted in more than 9,800 patients being evacuated in the six days from 10 to 15 March and 11 trains making 31 journeys.

Also in 1915, from 22 April to 27 May, and during the second Battle of Ypres, 147 train journeys were necessary to evacuate over 42,000 patients. At that time 15 trains were in service.

Later in 1915, during the Battle of Loos, the evacuation of

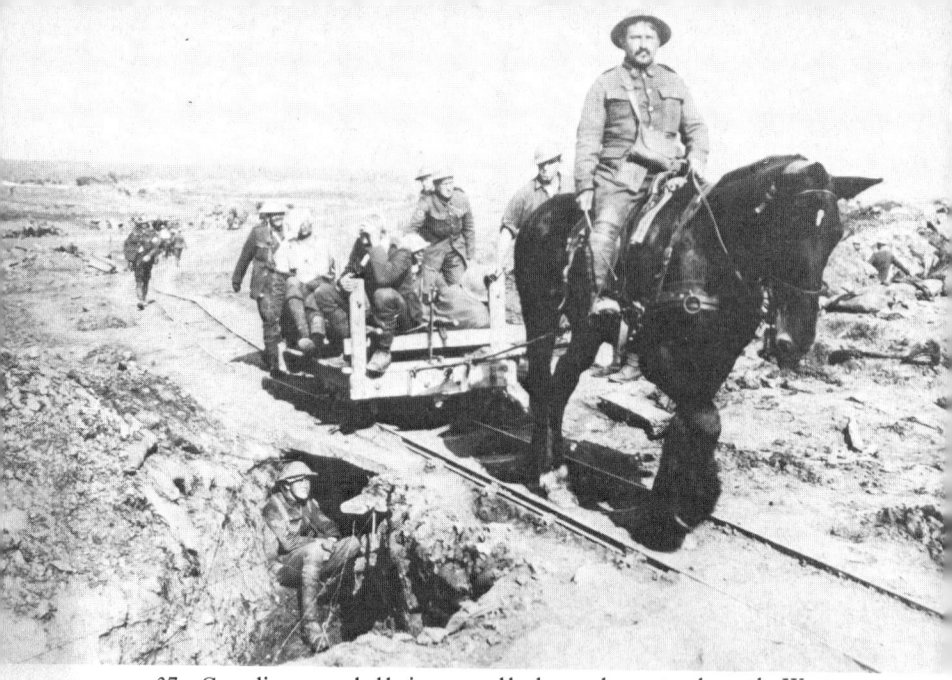

37 Canadian wounded being moved by horse-drawn trucks on the Western Front in 1916

22,390 casualties was carried out by 16 trains in 63 journeys.

But it was during the first Battle of the Somme that ambulance trains were used to their fullest capacity; in one period of four days, 1 to 4 July, 1916, 33,392 casualties were moved from rail-heads to bases on the coast in France. The magnitude of this operation can be appreciated from the statistical table in Appendix L.

Towards the end of 1917 three ambulance trains were sent to Italy (18, 22 and 24) and four more (21, 26, 30 and 31) soon followed. But they were found to be unsuitable for service there—especially on the very long haul from Taranto to the French ports, a distance of about 1,700 miles. (This route was used to avoid the sea route through the Straits of Gibraltar with the possibility of 'U' boat attacks on hospital ships.)

During 1918, with the exception of No 18, the trains were replaced by standard ambulance trains Nos 39, 41 and 43, all of which remained in Italy until after the end of the war. (No 41 was originally destined for Salonika but never got there because there was no crane strong enough at the port to unship eight-wheeled vehicles.) On 8 March, 1918, an Ambulance Train Depot and Supply Store, similar to that established in France a year earlier, was established at Arquata, north of Genoa.

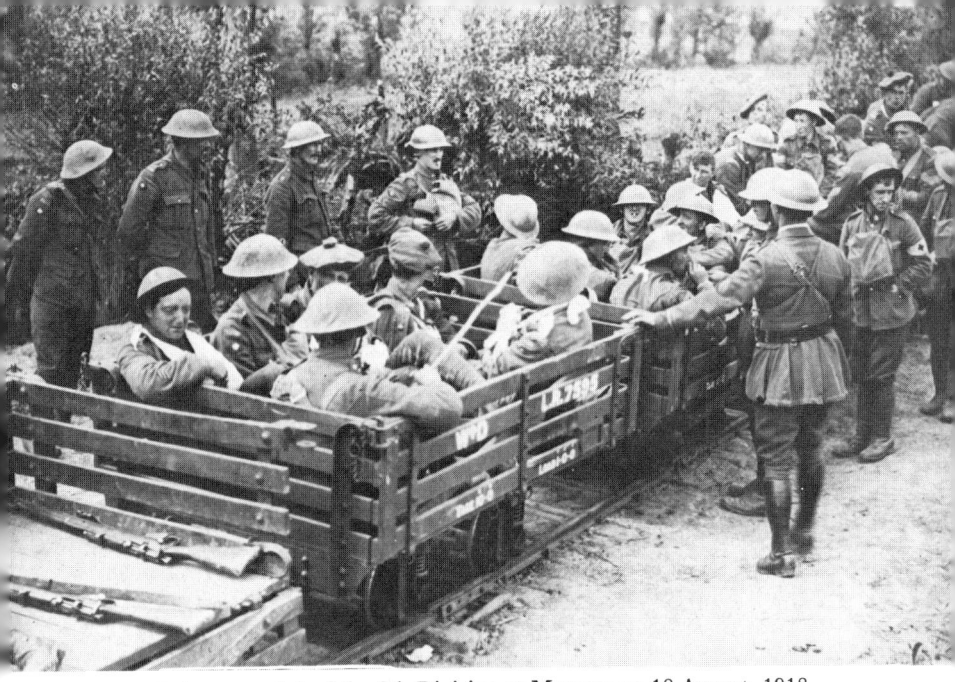

38 Sitting wounded of the 9th Division at Meteren on 18 August, 1918 during the Outtersteene ridge action

The British ambulance trains in Italy were on occasion supplemented by four temporary ambulance trains of the Italian State Railways. No 10 Italian Ambulance Train and an ambulance train of the Italian Maltese Order were also used for British patients; and among other Italian ambulance trains was the 'Rome Red Cross Special Ambulance Train'. In the spring of 1918 wounded were brought down from the Asiago Plateau by aerial railway to the British ambulance trains below.

Information about railway ambulance transport in other theatres of war and elsewhere is not available in such detail as that for France and Italy, but three ambulance trains were built in Egypt in 1914, and were staffed by RAMC personnel who had been mobilized in India and sent to Egypt for these units. Two more were constructed in Egypt in 1915, one of which was presented to the British Government by His Royal Highness Prince Yusef Kamel, President of the Egyptian Red Crescent Society. This train accommodated 12 officers and 96 other ranks, and was built in the Egyptian State railway workshops at a cost of £E 1,600.

Others were prepared or improvised for the Sinai Peninsula; these had to be lighter than normal trains, and two of them had LSWR coaches, each carrying seven stretchers on slings. Later the 'Bréchot-Déspres-Amelines' apparatus was used in these

119

trains. No 40 Ambulance Train, originally intended for Palestine, went to Egypt but was later relieved by another standard train. Other ambulance trains in Egypt were those numbered 44 to 51, and numbers 56 and 57.

On the narrow gauge Haifa-Damascus railway two trains were improvised by using the 'Zavodovski' method of carrying stretchers in slings.

On the Baghdad railway, another narrow gauge system, vehicles were improvised to carry 19 to 21 patients in bunks.

One of the trains constructed in India evacuated patients from Nasiriya to Basra, taking from eight to ten hours for the journey of just over 100 miles.

On the Dorian front in Macedonia the Decauville system was used in a train consisting of five open trucks. Four ambulance trains were also sent there from the United Kingdom and ambulance coaches were attached to supply trains. An improvised ambulance train was also used. It accommodated 50 lying patients, 12 on stretcher frames in one truck and 38 on the floor of seven other trucks. This train also had room for 240 sitting patients, 80 being carried in two third class coaches and 160 in eight trucks. The train had a staff of one medical officer and 11 other ranks.

Two Greek ambulance trains were based on Salonika and one was at the disposal of the British. This was an improvised train of ten covered trucks, and it used the 'Linxweiler' system of carrying stretchers on frames. In June, 1916, another improvised train was constructed using 24 carriages. This had a kitchen equipped with a Soyer's stove, a store and ration van, a van for the use of the medical officers which also served as an office, and one van for other rank personnel. In addition to ten passenger coaches it also had ten Greek ambulance vans—all of which were fitted with 'Bréchot-Déspres-Amelines' apparatus. Nos 52 and 53 Ambulance Trains were sent out from England in March, 1918. Another ambulance train was taken over from the Bulgarian authorities and used in this area, running to Sofia, Radomir and Dedeagach. It accommodated 50 lying and 120 sitting cases and carried a staff of one medical officer and 26 other ranks. In addition eight Decauville trains were in use.

A train of quite different character was the 'bath-train'. It was composed of 14 carriages and one 'bath' coach with 60 shower baths and was used at Jassy in Romania in 1916. The train was an experiment made by Dr de Forest, a member of one of the medical units of the Joint War Committee, sent out for service with the Servian Divisions in South Russia. At one time 1,800 troops bathed daily, their clothes being disinfected while they were doing so, and this undoubtedly checked the spread of typhus. The train was subsequently presented to the Romanians.

In Mesopotamia captured railway trucks were converted to carry 10 lying and 30 sitting patients, and railway ambulance trollies also carried patients on the railway lines. At one time a demand was made to the United Kingdom for five ambulance trains but only three appear to have been provided. Two of these were subsequently sub-divided into four trains which were numbered 1a, 1b, 2a and 2b. The third train found its way to Aden.

Nos 61 and 62 were among the medical units sent to Russia, where they were used on the Murmansk Railway. During the active operations on the railway systems in this area, troops were followed by a railway coach converted into a mobile dressing station.

An ambulance train accommodating both lying and sitting patients was organized at the base in Togoland, and the Catholic Mission at Lome helped to equip it. Rail transport was also used for ambulance purposes with the Western columns in the Cameroons. They appear to have been made up of six coaches, with 16 bunks in each coach.

In December, 1916, and during the early months of 1917, over 17,000 patients were carried on a 2 ft 6 inch gauge light railway at Kut-el-Amara.

Ambulance trains were also organized in East Africa on the Mombasa–Nairobi railway, while in South-West Africa an ambulance train was used on a Narrow-gauge railway.

The only railway ambulance transport available in South-West Africa, other than converted rolling stock was two of the coaches of the 'Princess Christian Hospital Train' which had been used in the South African War. Additional coaches of similar design were built and attached to the two old hospital train coaches, forming a new ambulance train. The South-African Railways also converted empty postal vans, putting in supports for stretchers, while at Bloemfontein an improvised ambulance train was organized by using the 'Zavodovski' method of carrying stretchers on slings in empty wagons. To deal with individual cases, a few motor-rail trollies were prepared and sent to the Northern and Central forces, but their use was very limited.

In Australia one of the Victoria Railway Company's 60 ft 'vestibule' express vans was converted to a hospital car to carry patients between Melbourne and Albury. There was accommodation for 12 ordinary patients in the larger ward, and for four infectious patients in a smaller ward.

In Canada passenger railway coaches were converted for the transportation of the more seriously wounded arriving at the eastern seaboard to hospitals and convalescent homes in the interior.

India, as we have already seen, had made preparations for the transport of patients by railway by having 'mock' ambulance trains on trial in peacetime. They were constructed by the Great Indian Peninsular Railway and were used on manoeuvres in the Poona District. Each train was made up of ten cars and was constructed so as to carry British and Indian patients in separate sectons of the train; they were staffed by British and Indian medical personnel.

Among the neutral countries of Europe, it is known that Sweden provided and staffed an ambulance train at Haparanda on the Russo—Swedish frontier, where Russian and German sick and wounded prisoners of war were exchanged.

When the United States of America entered the war in 1917 they ordered their ambulance trains from British railway companies. The first was provided in August of that year and by the end of the war 19 had been ordered. A further 29 were in course of construction when the armistice was signed. These 'USA' trains each carried 360 lying patients and had a staff of three medical officers, three nursing sisters and thirty orderlies. Details of their construction are included in Appendix M.

Altogether 63 ambulance trains were mobilized in the United

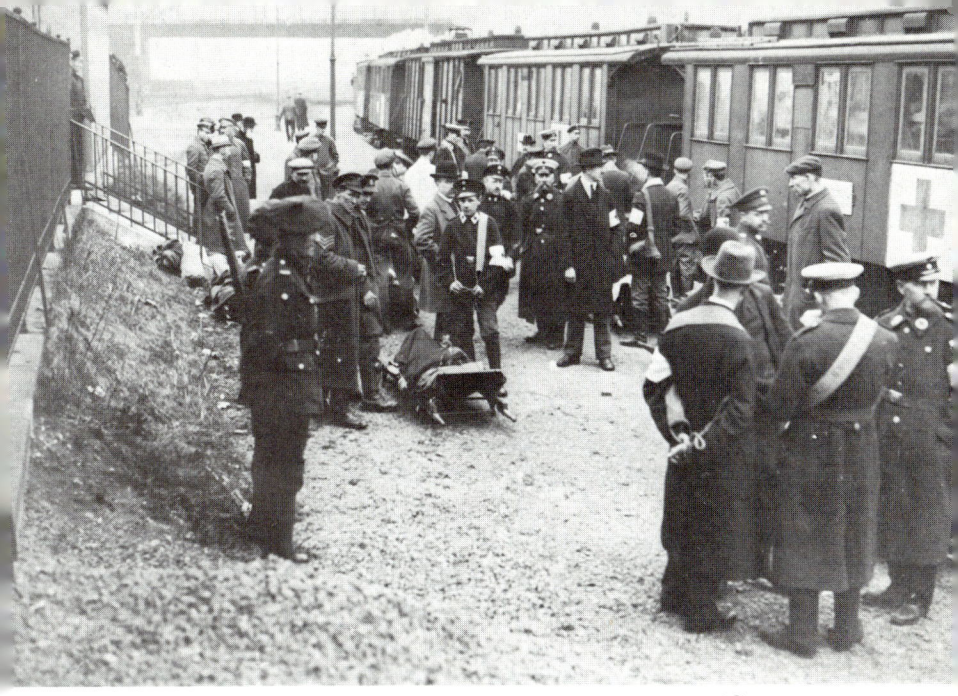

39 Repatriated German prisoners-of-war are transferred to No 15 German hospital train after their arrival in Cologne in March, 1919

Kingdom for the use of British forces and despatched to the various expeditionary forces overseas.

Some of the ambulance train rolling stock continued to be of service to the troops in France after the end of the war. During the post-armistice period an improvised Cologne Express was put into service to carry troops from Boulogne to Cologne. It was made up of ex-ambulance train carriages which provided ready-made sleeping accommodation on a journey of nearly 320 miles which, in those days, took about 19 hours. Later a number of similar trains were used as leave trains for the troops.

An aftermath of the First World War was the crisis in Turkey in 1922—the 'Chanak Affair'— when British troops were sent to Constantinople and other towns on both sides of the Dardanelles. A relief train was among the medical units provided by the British Red Cross Society, and was sent to alleviate the sufferings of the refugees. This train was loaded with tents, clothing, food and medical supplies and had four ambulance coaches—loaned by Her Royal Highness Princess Christian.

After the Quetta earthquake of 31 May, 1935, in which 23,000 people were killed, two ambulance trains were mobilized at Lahore and evacuated the seriously injured to Karachi, each train making two journeys. On an average seven passenger trains carrying the less badly injured were run from Quetta daily, while some of the British injured were similarly evacuated by passenger train, and others by air. The last ambulance train from there was on 18 June, 1935.

Statistics, although sometimes boring, can often convey a lot. In the Great War the British ambulance train service in France carried over 3,400,000 sick and wounded from the front to the bases, and more than 1,600,000 patients from base to base, a total of over five million patients carried between August, 1914, and December, 1918.

CHAPTER 10

Military Ambulance Trains in the United Kingdom in the First World War

The role of ambulance trains in the United Kingdom during the Great War differed completely from that of the trains overseas. Abroad, the patients were entrained, especially in France, from medical units scattered over an extensive area, often in the vicinity of the front line. In many cases their wounds and injuries only received emergency treatment, and often the patients still carried the mud and filth of the trenches. While in the train to the base they received proper attention and this was continued at the base hospitals and in the hospital ships and ambulance transports carrying them to the United Kingdom. Thus when they arrived at home ports they were in a presentable condition and only the seriously ill or badly wounded needed much medical attention on the next stage of their journey.

During the period 1897 to 1910 the War Railway Council dealt with the provision and equipping of ambulance trains on British railways in the event of war, and plans for the conversion of existing rolling stock were drawn up by the London and North Western Railway Company, in conjunction with the War Office medical authorities. The last modification to these plans was made in 1910 and complete drawings and specifications for the construction of ambulance trains were in existence by August, 1914.

On 25 August, 1914, Surgeon-General W. (later Sir William) Donovan, Army Medical Service was appointed Deputy Director of Medical Services, Southampton, with responsibility for the reception of the sick and wounded arriving in the United Kingdom. In 1917 the Embarkation Medical Service was

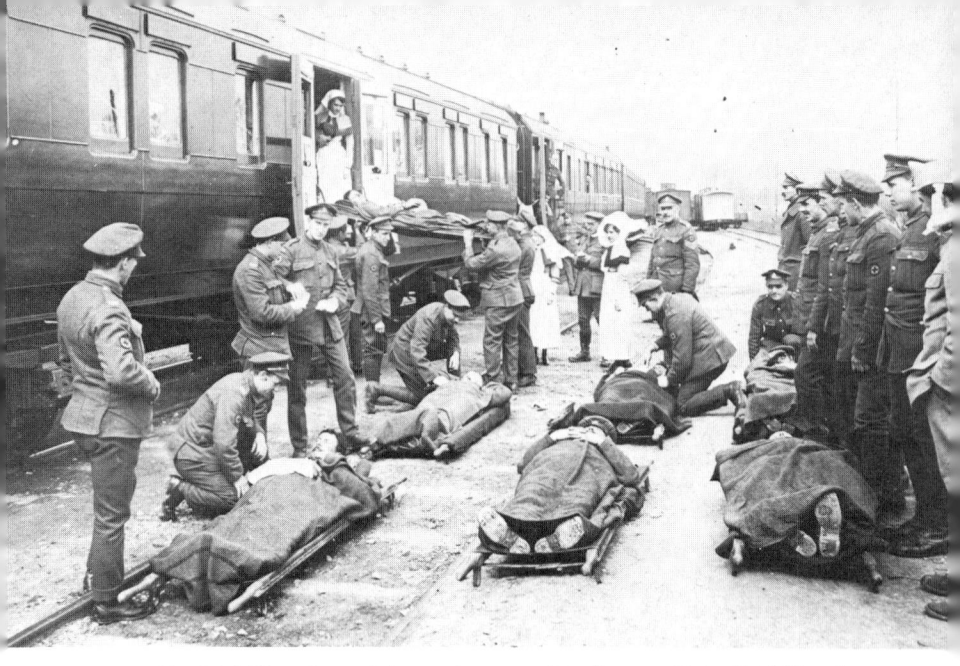

40 RAMC staff entraining patients near Doullens on 27 April, 1918 under the supervision of the sisters of the train

transferred to Adastral House, Thames Embankment, London, where Surgeon-General Donovan, then Director of Medical Services, Embarkation, continued in command.

The War Department Ambulance Train ('Netley Coaches') used during the South African War to carry patients arriving at Southampton to the Royal Victoria Hospital, Netley which was about five miles away and had its own railway siding, had continued its function in peacetime and on the out-break of war it was permanently stationed at Southampton Docks.

Originally 12 ambulance trains were constructed by the various railway companies in the United Kingdom and all reached Southampton in the very early days of the war. Two came from the Great Central, one from the Great Eastern, two from the Great Western, three from the London and North Western, two from the Midland and one each from the Lancashire and Yorkshire and the London and South Western. The total cost was estimated at about £24,000. Their 'make up' is shown in Appendix O. Somewhat later four emergency trains were taken into use for sitting patients; these were made up of ordinary corridor stock, together with dining cars.

The railways of Ireland supplied two trains. Train No 13 came from the Great Western Railway (Ireland) with vehicles converted to War Office requirements at the Railway's works at Dundalk, while the other came from the Great Southern and Western Railway Company (Ireland) and was fitted up at Ichincore works from main line rolling stock. (This Company also built an ambulance car 44 ft long which carried at least three ordinary iron bedsteads bolted to the floor. Called a 'dual' railway carriage, it could be worked over all systems in Ireland.) The two Irish trains distributed over 12,000 patients in the Dublin area, after they had arrived by hospital ship up the River Liffey.

There were also a number of North Eastern Railway Company vans which were fitted up for ambulance use. They were intended to be coupled to ordinary passenger trains for the carriage of any sick and wounded who had been disembarked on the north-east coast, and would take them to hospitals at Selby and York. The vans were lit by hurricane lamps and had red crosses painted on the outside. Large upper panels folded back on to the side of the wagon and an extremely wide ramp allowed the easy loading of 12 stretchers into each wagon.

The early 'home' ambulance trains had red crosses painted on the roofs as well as the sides of the carriage but they retained their companies' 'Liveries' and could thus be easily identified. Both the Great Central and the Great Eastern were varnished teak, while the Lancashire and Yorkshire train had brown upper panels and maroon lower panels. The London and North Western was more distinctive with bluish-white above and a purple-brown below. The London and South Western, which had upper panels and mouldings of a salmon shade of pink, contrasted with the cream and crimson-lake of the Great Western and the South Eastern and Chatham's overall brown. The Midland colours were crimson-lake lined with yellow, while the Great Western (Ireland) was varnished on either mahogany or teak. The Great Southern and Western (Ireland) had purple-lake sides lined out in yellow and red. Not to be outdone, the War Department Ambulance Train had its own distinctive 'livery' and this is described in Appendix P.

When Dover was brought into use as a reception port for the sick and wounded from the BEF in 1915, a number of ambulance trains were permanently transferred there from Southampton. These two ports merit special mention.

On the outbreak of war Southampton became No 1 Military Embarkation Port and practically the whole port was taken over by the military authorities. From here the entire British Expeditionary Force was despatched to France over the short period 9 to 31 August, 1914. The first convoy home, carrying 111 sick and wounded reached Southampton on 24 August, 1914, and the patients were taken in the War Department Ambulance Train to the Royal Victoria Hospital, Netley, some London and South Western passenger coaches being added for the sitting patients. The first regular ambulance train to make a journey was the Great Central, which took 62 lying and 125 sitting patients to Netley four days later. On 29 August the Lancashire and Yorkshire train received a convoy of 65 lying and 121 sitting cases from the hospital ship *St Andrew* and took them to Well Hall, Kent. All casualties which were evacuated from France in 1914 were disembarked at Southampton, one of the highly appreciated features of this port being that it had an exceptionally large boiler plant which could simultaneously heat eight ambulance trains on separate sidings.

The new Marine station at Dover was not completed when the war started but the suitability of Dover as a reception port for hospital ships was soon recognized. By the end of 1914 the station had been sufficiently prepared for the transfer of patients from ship to train. When the port became fully operational in 1915 it was possible for two hospital ships and six ambulance trains to be dealt with at the same time.

The total number of home ambulance trains in service eventually reached 29, of which 24 (with a peak carrying capacity of 8,412) were for the Army, the remainder being for the Navy. Additional emergency trains were made up when required, with vans to take lying patients on stretchers while corridor coaches were attached for sitting patients. These trains, which were provided with a kitchen car, accommodated from 300 to 500 patients.

Fairly early in the war Major R. W. D. Leslie introduced his own system of improvisation—the 'trestle' system—because the established systems such as the 'Zavodovski' and the 'Bréchot-Déspres-Amelines' were found to have certain faults, while other systems did not make full use of all available space, or else they needed costly structural alterations or special metal fittings which were not readily available. The 'trestle' system was simplicity itself—just a matter of supporting stretchers on moveable wooden trestles in vestibule vans. Patients were able to be loaded and unloaded with practically the same speed as in regular ambulance trains; no structural alterations were necessary, no metal fittings were needed—and full use was made of all available space. The trestles themselves were made of wood, and when folded, a pair (which could easily be carried by one orderly) needed little storage space. Two trains were made up to use this system—the London and North Western Railway providing 42 ft vestibule vans, while the London and South Western made the trestles. Each van had overhead lighting and adequate ventilation, and accommodated 20 stretchers. These emergency trains proved their worth when additional accommodation was needed to deal with patients from the larger hospital ships, such as when the *Aquitania, Britannic* and *Mauretania* disembarked their thousands of patients from Gallipoli.

The distribution of patients after their arrival in the United Kingdom was a complicated undertaking. Their destination depended to a large extent on the nature of their disability—it being essential that certain cases should go to hospitals specializing in particular types of treatment. Australian, Canadian and New Zealand casualties, however, usually went to hospitals which their own medical personnel had established in Britain; and German prisoners-of-war had to be sent to special P.O.W. hospitals. To facilitate distribution, advance information was cabled about the various categories of patients on each hospital ship and the estimated time of arrival. In addition to stating the totals of lying and sitting patients, these categories were sub-divided into the numbers of officers, nurses and other ranks, with further sub-divisions into surgical, medical, infectious, mental, and any other special cases.

Patients on the hospital ships were also labelled with one of five areas corresponding to their home area—London and Southern; West of England; Midlands; North England and Scotland; Ireland. Thus there was always a possibility that patients could be sent to a hospital in the vicinity of their home.

Daily notification was sent by the area home commands showing the bed situation in their larger and specialist hospitals.

Before disembarkation began, the huge sheds which separated hospital ships at their berths and ambulance trains in the sidings were lit and heated. These sheds were about a quarter of a mile in length, and while awaiting entrainment lying patients were accommodated in smaller heated enclosures.

Officers and nursing sisters were the first patients to be disembarked, the former usually being sent to London in the War Department Ambulance Train. Then one train after another pulled into the shed—those which had the longest journeys to make being loaded first. All hospital ships were cleared on the day on which disembarkation began and this occasionally meant that some trains had to make double journeys.

Generally the patients had received adequate medical attention before being disembarked and, except for emergency treatment, there was little for the medical officers and nursing sisters to do, other than to replace soiled dressings and administer medicines. The staff of the trains made out the usual nominal rolls, did the normal ward duties and prepared and supplied hot drinks and light refreshments. It was important to ensure that each patient always had his 'dorothy-bag'. Many of the stretcher cases were only clad in pyjamas, and their 'dorothy-bags' were the sole receptacle for those personal odds and ends which in many cases had sustained them in the line, such as letters from home, photographs, possibly a few French francs, an unused 'green envelope', an odd souvenir and other items.

When the war began there were about 7,000 beds in military hospitals in the United Kingdom. The larger military hospitals, which received the earliest convoys of sick and wounded, were the Alexandra Hospital, Cosham; the Cambridge and Connaught Hospitals, Aldershot; The Queen Alexandra Military Hospital, Millbank; the Royal Herbert Hospital, Woolwich; and the Royal Victoria Hospital, Netley. Smaller military hospitals were located at Chatham, Chester, Colchester, Devonport, Edinburgh, Shorncliffe, Tidworth and York. In

Ireland there were hospitals at Belfast, Cork, the Curragh and Dublin.

By May, 1915, the RAMC Territorial Force had mobilized general hospitals at Aberdeen, Birmingham, Brighton, Bristol, Cambridge, Cardiff, Leeds, Leicester, Lincoln, Liverpool, London, Manchester, Newcastle-on-Tyne, Oxford, Plymouth, Portsmouth and Sheffield. Many civilian institutions and premises, such as hospitals, asylums, infirmaries, schools and university buildings, were requisitioned for the treatment of war casualties.

The larger hospitals distributed their patients when they were fit to travel, to smaller military, civilian, auxiliary and private hospitals and to convalescent homes; many, too, were sent home on sick leave, and thus accommodation was made available for incoming convoys.

In June, 1916, there were 200,000 beds available for service patients. This figure rose to 300,000 in 1917, and at the time of the armistice had reached 364,133.

Nearly 200 railway stations in Britain received convoys of sick and wounded; Strathpeffer in Scotland, 624 miles from Southampton, was the most distant.

To properly appreciate the task of the embarkation medical authorities it again helps to include some statistics. The total number of British and Commonwealth sick and wounded dealt with at all ports in the United Kingdom during the period August, 1914, to August, 1920, exceeded 2,655,000—the number of sick being slightly in excess of the wounded. In addition, some 14,000 Indian, 8,500 American and 900 Belgian patients, and more than 27,500 sick and wounded German and Austrian prisoners-of-war were disembarked.

From 24 August, 1914, to 31 December, 1918, ambulance trains made 7,822 journeys from Southampton, distributing over 1,250,000 patients. During the Gallipoli campaign in 1915 the *Aquitania* berthed with nearly 5,000 sick and wounded; it took 20 ambulance trains to transfer them to hospitals at home.

The figures for Dover cover the period from 2 January, 1915 to 28 February, 1919, during which approximately 1,260,000 patients were received. It needed over 4,000 hospital ship journeys to bring them to port and almost 7,800 ambulance train journeys were required to distribute them to home hospitals. Dover's busiest time was in April, 1918, when upwards of 66,000 casualties were disembarked from 229 hospital ships. They were distributed throughout the United Kingdom by 372 ambulance trains, which ran at an average of over 12 a day.

Other ports were also used for the reception of sick and wounded. About 23,000 patients from the Mediterranean area were disembarked at Avonmouth, while Devonport, Liverpool and Tilbury received patients from the Far East. Those from North Russia were sent to Leith and many repatriated sick and wounded prisoners-of-war dealt with at Boston, Folkestone, Hull, Newcastle and the Port of London, while about 12,000 went direct to Ireland, mainly for transfer to hospitals in the Dublin area.

Mention was made in the previous chapter of the fact that over 33,000 patients were moved in France from railheads at the front during the first Battle of the Somme. The ramifications of that tragedy are illustrated by the fact that during the week ending 9 July, 1916, 151 ambulance trains left Southampton with more than 30,000 patients—the maximum being on 9 July, when 29 trains took away over 6,000 patients. During the whole period of this battle, 117,000 casualties reached the United Kingdom—68,000 at Southampton and 49,000 at Dover.

CHAPTER 11

Naval Ambulance Trains in the United Kingdom in the First World War

There is not the same detailed information available about Naval ambulance trains which did duty in the United Kingdom as there is for trains used by the Army. However, certain details are of special interest because they show essential differences between the trains used by the two services.

The main difference was that the early Naval trains had moveable cots, whereas Army trains had fixed beds. The Naval medical authorities decided on the moveable cot system for three reasons. It allowed a patient to be placed in a 'medical service' cot in his own ship or in a Naval hospital ship, to then be carried in that cot to an ambulance train and subsequently remain in the same cot when transferred to a Naval hospital. On all occasions replacement cots—complete with mattress, blankets and pillow—were handed over for those which carried patients. The use of such a cot therefore obviated the continual transfer of patients from stretcher to bed and vice versa. Under the fixed-bed Army system the bed and its patient also became a component part of the ambulance coach and were thus subject to every movement when running. This was reduced to a minimum when the Naval moveable cot was used.

Naval ambulance cots were constructed of canvas stretched over a flat wooden frame. The two ends of the canvas formed a triangle, in the apex of which was an eye-piece for the insertion of a rope or lanyard. The cot contained a hair mattress, two blankets and a pillow. The canvas sides of the cot extended sufficiently to enable them to be brought over and fixed to the other side by pins. The sides could also be laced up at each end, so that the patient could be in an enclosed 'box'. This was essential, for casualties in naval vessels very frequently have to be slung over the side of the ship to be transferred to hospital ships at sea, or removed from fighting or hospital ships on reaching port. However, while only two bearers are needed to carry army patients on stretchers, four are required to carry naval cots to an ambulance train, and two more to fix the cots to the hooks in the roof of the ward cars.

Naval ambulance trains had their cots slung in two tiers of twelve on each side of the ward coach. The upper cots were suspended directly from two hooks in the coach roof; the lower ones were suspended from the same hooks by the use of a lanyard fitted with an eye at the upper end and a hook at the lower. The lanyards, which were of standard length, were interchangeable and could also be used for slinging stretchers, or for suspending special cot cases in the centre of the coach. When the cots were in position they were firmly lashed to the sides of the coach—a 'fender' being placed between the cot framework and the coach side. Lateral movement was absorbed by this fender, while vertical jolting was practically eliminated by suspension. The fenders were made of canvas-covered pads of tow, mounted on wooden bases and screwed to the sides of the coach.

In the middle of 1915 the naval medical authorities tried another suspension method of carrying patients, which was designed to combine the advantages of the naval moveable cot and of the army fixed bed. It was also considered to have advantages of its own, and was termed the 'gripe' suspension system. (In nautical vocabulary 'gripe' is the tendency of a vessel under sail to head up into the wind.) It used beds made of rectangular frames of light tubular steel—6 ft by 1 ft 9 ins—across which a spring mattress was stretched in the ordinary manner. The frames of the bed were supported by placing them in four hooks which were lined with a rubber pad. The hooks were attached to chains suspended from the roof of the coach. The bed was kept in position and prevented from lateral movement by means of a 'gripe' which was hooked on to the centre of the frame on the gangway side and passed underneath the bed. The 'gripe' consisted of two pieces of light chain coupled with a special spring of appropriate tension.

On the outbreak of war two ambulance trains were provided for the Admiralty, a further three being added later. The first was completed by the North British Railway Company on 7 August, 1914; it had 96 cots and was used in Scotland throughout the war. A second was delivered by the London and North Western Railway Company on 8 August, 1914, and went to Chatham dockyard. Nos 3 and 4 came into use in June, 1916, while No 5 did not operate until March, 1918. Both 4 and 5 were constructed by the South Eastern and Chatham Railway Company and they were used to carry Naval patients on the steep gradients of Scottish railways. The same company also provided two emergency ambulance trains very early in the war, each made up of 11 vehicles, of which nine were passenger carriages for sitting patients. These trains made several trips, but one was released in September, 1914, and the other in December.

Naval ambulance trains were manned like warships, watches being kept by day and night. The 'port' and 'starboard' side of each train was referred to and the letters and figures were appropriately red and green. The exteriors were painted 'navy grey' with red crosses on white backgrounds.

The North British train spent two and a half years at Inverness, entraining patients at Invergordon and taking them to Edinburgh or as far north as Thurso. It also took patients from Port Edgar on the Forth to Wemyss Bay on the west coast, and from Larbert to Edinburgh.

Four naval ambulance trains worked between Scotland and England—two being stabled at Edinburgh, one at Glasgow and one at Chatham. The trains from Edinburgh made a fixed weekly tour calling as required at ports on the east coast and then going to Chatham, Gosport and Plymouth.

There was always one train at Chatham—the train which arrived one week remaining until the next week's train arrived. On their return journeys these trains serviced Greenwich, London and Southend, removing convalescent patients to other naval hospitals. From Southend they travelled to Willesden Junction to pick up convalescent officers who had travelled there from Plymouth or Portsmouth by ordinary passenger train. These trains then moved on to Peebles.

The train stationed at Glasgow journeyed south via Larbert and Edinburgh, and a supplementary train also made a weekly trip from Edinburgh to the south; in addition there was always one train on 'stand-by' for emergency use.

Naval ambulance trains worked the Highland Railway route from Invergordon on an average of one a week, making a total of 208 journeys from 1915 to 1918. During the same period, over 1200 calls were made at various stations on the North British Railway, and more than 600 on Caledonian Railway stations.

Independent of those brought direct to Chatham, Plymouth and Portsmouth, the number of patients carried by naval ambulance trains totalled 77,781—of whom 27,148 were cot cases and the remaining 50,633 were sitting patients. It should be realized that sick men are not wanted on fighting ships at all—indeed there is no room for them. Unless they are likely to effect a speedy and complete recovery it is in the best interests of all concerned that they be evacuated as quickly as possible and replaced by fit men.

Originally there were two types of naval ambulance trains —the larger accommodating 136 cot cases and the smaller having room for only 40 lying patients, but taking 36 sitting cases as well. The normal complement of the larger trains was two medical officers and 36 sick-berth ratings. Nursing sisters did duty on the trains when their services were necessary.

Details of the make up of No 1 Naval Ambulance Train are in Appendix Q. Up to the end of 31 December, 1914, this train had travelled more than 8,000 miles with over 1,700 patients of various categories—Army, Belgian, German as well as Navy. The maximum number taken on one journey was 363.

Like the Army, the Navy also exhibited one of their ambulance trains for fund-raising purposes in June, 1916, at Addison Road, Kensington and the receipts from the admission fee of 1/– were donated to the Dreadnought Seamen's Hospital at Greenwich. The Army frequently exhibited at stations and raised over £5,000.

Before beginning the next chapter, let us recall two naval engagements—the Battle of Jutland and Zeebrugge.

Most of the casualties from the Battle of Jutland which

started on 31 May, 1916, arrived at Invergordon, Port Edgar and Rosyth on board the hospital ships to which they had been transferrred from the fighting vessels. Some patients went direct to nearby hospitals while others were taken by naval ambulance trains to more distant destinations. Two trains received casualties direct from the naval hospital ships which arrived at Invergordon; the first left the port at 9.34 pm on 3 June and the second at 8.12 pm the following day. Between them they carried 554 naval casualties, and all were accommodated in hospital within a couple of days of the end of the engagement.

The Zeebrugge operations of April, 1918, made naval history, and naval ambulance trains played their part in the way in which they distributed the casualties. The operations started at an early hour in the morning of 23 April, 1918, on which date No 3 Naval Ambulance Train went to Chatham to receive casualties and take them to Chatham naval hospital. The first patients arrived on HMS *Vindictive,* and their entrainment started at 9.50 am, being completed in less than one and a half hours. Apart from two serious cases who were sent to the military hospital at Dover, and some slightly wounded who went to Deal, the remaining 150 went in the train to Chatham and arrived there at 1.38 pm. To deal with the arrival of further casualties, No 5 Naval Ambulance Train had left Edinburgh the previous night and it reached Dover at 12.30 pm, just as the *Daffodil* came alongside with one lying and three sitting casualties. Then two more cases were taken off HMS *Arrogant* and at 2.45 pm the *Iris* arrived with 84 more. All these patients were entrained by 4.25 pm, and were off-loaded at Chatham by 5.42 pm. So altogether some 200 naval officers and ratings who had been wounded in the early hours of the morning off the Belgian coast were brought across the channel by various vessels, landed at Dover, put into naval ambulance trains and admitted to hospital at Chatham on the late afternoon of the same day.

CHAPTER 12

Military Ambulance Trains in the United Kingdom and Overseas in the Second World War

Detailed information about ambulance trains which were used at home and overseas in the Second World War is, strangely, not so readily available as for the First World War, and this chapter must therefore be of a more general nature.

Before hostilities began, the authorities had decided that 12 ambulance trains would be immediately required, eight for the United Kingdom and four to go overseas with the expeditionary force. Detailed designs and drawings had been prepared by the London, Midland and Scottish Railway, vehicles selected from their stock and the appropriate fittings assembled at Derby. Instructions for their construction were issued on 2 September, 1939, when the selected vehicles were distributed to the four railway groups in existence at that time; the Great Western; the London, Midland and Scottish; the London and North Eastern and the Southern, each of which constructed its own quota of trains. In less than three weeks two home and four overseas trains were handed over to the military authorities.

By October, however, it was apparent that many more trains would be needed and an Ambulance Train Committee composed of members of the Armed Forces, the Ministry of Transport and representatives from the Railway Groups was constituted; it was responsible for the supply of ambulance trains and the maintenance of rolling stock. The London, Midland and Scottish Railway acted as the link between the government departments, the Railway Executive Committee and the four Railway Groups.

By the spring of 1940 25 ambulance trains had been constructed; 12 for home use and 13 for service overseas, a procedure which involved the conversion of 344 London, Midland and Scottish vehicles. In August, 1942, a further 23 trains were requisitioned for use by the Allied Forces overseas, and later orders raised the total to 66. Each railway group converted its own rolling stock to provide these trains. In addition, the War Organization of the British Red Cross Committee provided four home ambulance trains whose design comformed with that of the Ambulance Train Committee.

The ambulance trains required for use in the United Kingdom were originally made up of nine varying types of vehicles; two more coaches were added later. As in the earlier war these trains had the usual ward coaches for lying as well as sitting patients, with separate accommodation for mental and other special patients. They included a kitchen car, a vehicle for use as a pharmacy, office and medical store and living compartments for medical officers, nursing sisters and other rank personnel.

Much later in the war, ambulance trains were needed for the American Forces in the United Kingdom and the first, which was made up of Great Western rolling stock, was handed over on 25 March, 1943. This company constructed special sidings on the north of the main line at Shrivenham, Wiltshire, for the reception of American casualties. Ten North Eastern engines were specially allotted to run these trains and two crews of drivers, together with firemen, fitters and guards were provided by the same company to operate the trains, on which they lived with the American medical personnel. A 14-coach ambulance train for an American ambulance train maintenance unit was also constructed by the Great Western and was stabled at Swindon. Similar but smaller provision was made for British troops, and four coaches were prepared on 6 June, 1944, for No 1 Railway Workshop Company, Royal Engineers.

The Americans were also supplied with five LSWR '1905 vintage' stock railway coaches which were converted into selfcontained railway ambulance cars for the movement of small numbers of patients. Like the coaches of the old 'War Department Ambulance Train', they were stabled at the Royal Victoria Hospital, Netley, which had been handed over to the USA on the entry of America into the war. These coaches accommodated 24 lying and 12 sitting patients and had the usual cooking and toilet facilities.

At the end of hostilities they were transferred to the Longmoor Military Railway and subsequently loaned to British Railways for use on their special trains carrying pilgrims to Lourdes.

Before the outbreak of war the French Government had offered four of their ambulance trains for the use of the British Forces in their country; they said that they would be ready for service within three weeks of the outbreak of war. Two were *'trains-couché'* each of which accommodated 300 lying patients and the others were *'trains-mixte'* which only had room for 120 cot cases but accommodated 240 sitting patients as well. But there is no record that these trains were ever taken into use.

The thirteen ambulance trains for France were transported by ferry from Southampton and Harwich to Calais. All had red crosses on a white ground painted on their roofs as well as on their sides, but this did not protect them from enemy attack. In France they were divided into two groups; one group operated in the forward area and was thus liable to encounter the enemy at close quarters. The second group based further south and was consequently able to continue in service until the Dunkirk evacuation. Nine ambulance trains were lost in the early months of the war, but the remaining four were stabled somewhere in France, and were brought back into service in 1944.

By the end of the war British Railways had converted over 900 railway vehicles into 74 ambulance trains for the British and American forces. Another 32 were under construction when the war ended, and there was a request on hand from the Americans for an additional 45.

Once again a few illuminating statistics: during the evacuation of the BEF from Dunkirk and other French ports, which covered the period from the end of May until 10 June, 1940, over 31,000 service casualties were carried in 47 ambulance train journeys and subsequently admitted to military and Emergency Medical Service hospitals in the United Kingdom.

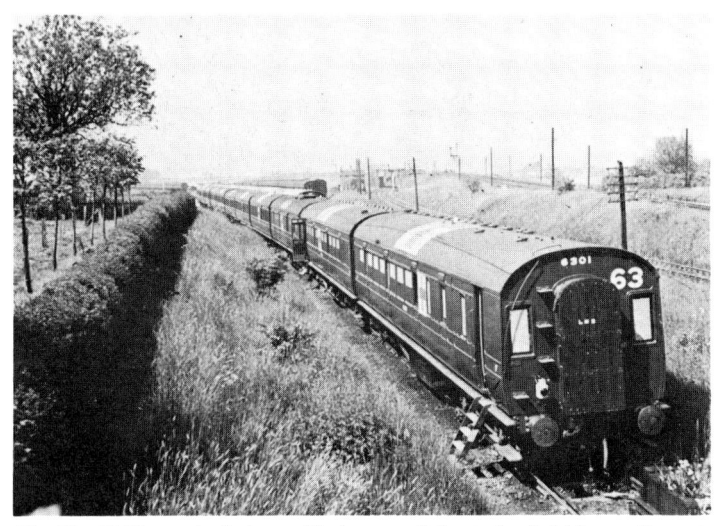

41 No 63 Home Ambulance Train-one of the trains held in readiness to receive casualties from overseas. It was one of the four home ambulance trains presented to the British Government by the British Red Cross Society-Order of St John

From the D-day operations on, 6 June, 1944, to 8 May, 1945, over 1,800 ambulance train journeys with patients were made in the United Kingdom. As in the earlier war, Southampton was the leading port for the reception of casualties, and they were put on ambulance trains at Southampton Docks, Southampton Terminus, Gosport, Netley, Cosham, Ringwood, Stockbridge, and other nearby railway stations. The first invasion casualties arrived on 7 June, 1944, and in that month there were 104 train journeys, each with about 300 patients; in July the number of journeys had risen to 113. The total number of patients carried during this entire period approximated to 360,000.

On 15 September, 1944, the first party of repatriated sick and wounded prisoners of war arrived at the Clyde; four ambulance trains and one ordinary train were required to distribute them to hospitals in the U.K.

It is again necessary to deal separately with the transport of naval casualties. In the early days they were moved under arrangements made by a central movements control which

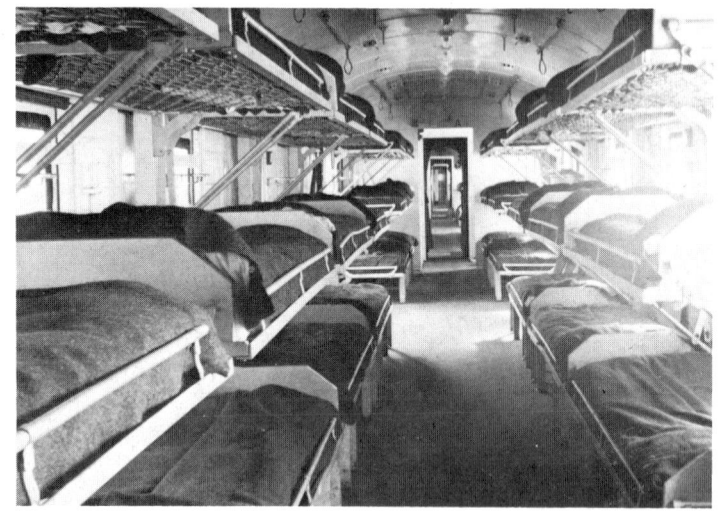

42 The interior of ward coach A3 of No 63 Home Ambulance Train

dealt with all service and civilian casualties. But in 1944, during the invasion of Normandy, all ambulance trains and civilian evacuation trains were under the direct control of the War Office and there was a problem when dealing with naval patients. While army and air force invalids travelled with the minimum of baggage which could be carried in luggage compartments attached to ambulance trains, the naval patients were at a great disadvantage, for they had to travel with their bags and hammocks, 'ditty' boxes, private suitcases and other bulky impedimenta which at times caused delay and dislocated plans. Eventually special baggage accommodation had to be provided when naval patients were to be entrained.

There were, however, two instances where rail ambulance coaches were specially converted and used for naval medical transport which were not under the Central Movements Control of the Ministry of Health or of the War Office. Two North Eastern Railway Company vans were converted to take 24 stretcher cases each on supporting racks; two brake 'third' vans from the same company were adapted to carry 6 lying and 24 sitting patients. These four vehicles were made up into two units which had one of each type of van with a total carrying capacity of 30 lying and 24 sitting patients. They were stabled at Waverley Station, Edinburgh, and attached to passenger trains on their routine runs between Edinburgh and Aberdeen. The vans were heated and had facilities for serving hot drinks and light meals.

During 1942 a rail ambulance coach was stabled at Bristol; it was a 57 ft composite railway restaurant car specially converted for naval medical transport purposes. The original galley was retained in the centre of the car but the third class dining compartment was stripped and converted into a small ward for light cot cases.

At least 14 ambulance trains and three ambulance coaches appear to have been used in the Burma campaign. At the beginning of December, 1941, two trains were made up of converted first and second class coaches of the Burma Railway—the gauge of the track being one metre. Seven were Indian ambulance trains. Some were based at Chittagong, Debrugarh, Manipur Road and Silchar but no details of their journeys are known. Some did, however, travel on the Bengal Assam Railway to Manipur Road and Ledo. On the withdrawal from Burma, No 2 (Burma) Ambulance Train—with five extra coaches attached—entrained 438 patients together with 73 of the staff of medical units. It made its journey in two parts—at a stop outside Mandalay the train crews simply disappeared. New crews were obtained and after a five-day journey an airfield was reached from where the patients and the nursing officers were evacuated by air to India.

India produced 31 ambulance trains and similar rail transport during the war. Of these 14 were for broad-gauge tracks, 13 for one metre tracks and one for a narrow track. Three standard trains were constructed for overseas use—while personnel were provided for train duty in Persia, Iraq and Ceylon. In addition there were independent ward coaches which could carry from 16 to 25 patients and smaller ambulance coaches which had room for only 14 patients, who were carried for very short distances.

In the Abyssinian and Somaliland campaigns four ambulance trains were converted from local rolling stock, each taking 76 stretcher cases. Extra coaches were added for 'sitters', the maximum load carried by any one train being 320. Two of these trains were based at Gebeit, the others at Khartoum. In addition, the staffs of two ambulance transports converted railway sleeping cars for the evacuation of small numbers of patients for entrainment in the ambulance trains. Subsequently these coaches were joined together to form a fifth train.

There were nine ambulance trains in North-West Africa, five British and four French. A number of Michelin Diesel Auto-Rail cars were obtained from the French—these providing an average daily lift of 160 patients in almost equal numbers of lying and sitting patients.

The ambulance train story of Italy is rather vague. A service composed of ambulance trains built out of ordinary rolling stock ran between Bari and Taranto, and Termoli and Bari. Originally there were four but two were withdrawn, one because it was badly damaged, while the other went on the Naples line of communication. Nine ambulance trains were used in the clearance of patients from hospitals in Rome at the beginning of July. In August, Nos 1 (Egyptian), 2, 6, 70 and 71 were disbanded, the last four being reformed as numbers 77, 78, 79 and 80.

In North Russia ambulance trains ran regularly between Murmansk and Archangel. The entire journey by train took five to six days, but when the Beloye Gulf was crossed by sea the train journey took only about 12 hours.

There was no No 13 Ambulance Train in France in the First World War—but there must have been less superstition in the Second World War. No 13's particular story began on 15 May, 1940, when it was awaiting orders outside Lille, well within the battle zone. Convoys of patients arrived from various casualty clearing stations in the afternoon; there were 170 stretcher cases and each had to be carried over two railway tracks and down a long platform to be loaded on to the train. There were other patients as well, some just released from hospital while others were convalescing; there were also some seriously wounded Belgians. When all had been entrained, No 13 moved into Lille where more patients were waiting to be taken on.

They were mostly serious cases and had arrived at the train direct from a casualty clearing station, in many cases only being dressed with a First Field Dressing. By 1 am there were 350 patients on board, including some French wounded and five German officers. The latter displayed such arrogance that they were detrained at the first opportunity so that members of their own medical service could take care of them. The train arrived at St Omer at 6 am the next morning and went towards Calais an hour later. Calais, however, was under heavy bombardment; the harbour was practically out of action and the railway tracks were broken up. After a wait of several hours the train moved on, bypassing Boulogne, to Étaples. By this time the enemy were only eight miles away, and the station-master told the Commanding Officer that the station was about to be blown up. So No 13 moved on to Boulogne; but as this was under air attack the train moved 20 miles back to Dannes-Camies. Here some German wounded were unloaded and, to the delight of the patients, some cigarettes and chocolates were taken on board. At 1 am the train made a second visit to Boulogne —which was then quiet. That was Wednesday 22 May. No 13 had been on the move for the best part of a week, always in the area of enemy operations.

Next is the story of No 3 Ambulance Train. In the first week of the battle of Flanders—May, 1940—it stopped at a small railway station with the advancing enemy only four miles away. The convoy of wounded which was to be entrained had not got through, but about 50 refugees were taken on board and moved to a safer place. The train then went to Verneuil where it had been ascertained that a convoy of patients would be waiting. By the time ten patients had been entrained, No 3 found itself in the middle of an enemy air attack. Fortunately an ammunition train on a nearby line had just been moved before the raid began but there was a French troop train alongside. When the raid was over it was found that No 5 coach was like a crumpled matchbox, some of the other coaches were tilted over and broken glass and earth covered the train. The French troop train was in ruins. In the evening the patients and staff got away in the first three coaches leaving the body of one orderly who had been killed under the wreckage of the train.

A third story concerns No 4 Ambulance Train, again in May, 1940. On the 10th of that month the train was at a village just outside Dieppe with a staff of five medical officers, three nursing sisters and 40 orderlies. Trouble started a few days later when, at Nivose, it was entraining casualties from a casualty clearing station, which, because of the intense air activity had to be evacuated. This enemy air activity continued throughout the period the patients were being taken on board the train. Some of the medical officers and other staff were also transferred from the casualty clearing station to this ambulance train.

Its departure from Nivose was undertaken with the greatest difficulty, firstly because the Belgian railway system had lapsed into a state of chaos and secondly because the Belgian engine driver refused to take the train out of Belgium. The Commanding Officer soon solved the latter problem; he put an armed guard of two men in the driver's cabin and the engine driver decided to move on. The second problem was that the signals were against the train, so the Commanding officer got out of the train and changed them, a procedure which he repeated about a dozen times, until the train was out of Belgium. Dieppe was reached on 18 May, after the train had been missing for the best part of a week. Like other missing trains it was thought to have been lost, and its staff made prisoners of war.

On the next day the patients were distributed among the General Hospitals in Dieppe. The day after, because of intense bombing, the staff took refuge under the train.

By 21 May No 4 Ambulance Train was doing its job again, evacuating patients from Nos 1 and 10 General Hospitals, and also from an Indian General Hospital at Dieppe. Between 600 and 800 patients were taken on, many seriously wounded, and ten nursing sisters were also entrained. The train's engine was not forthcoming however, and while the train was waiting at Dieppe harbour siding a very heavy air raid took place. Two hospital ships, the *Maid of Kent* and the *Brighton*, and a tanker, were lying close by at the dockside. The tanker was soon on fire and it quickly spread to the *Maid of Kent* and the *Brighton*. Then No 4 Ambulance Train began to burn. The walking cases ran to nearby shelters and were machine-gunned, many being killed. Part of the train became a raging inferno and the patients in one ward, some hobbling along in Thomas's splits and others with their heads swathed in bandages, advised the nursing sisters not to enter the coach which they thought had been gassed. Fortunately this was not so; all that had happened was that the fumes from the bombed tanker had filled the ward, all the windows of the train having been smashed. The fumes cleared fairly quickly and the patients were put back to bed. Many huge pieces of iron from the bombed tanker had passed right through the woodwork of the train from one side to the other but fortunately without wounding any of the patients or staff. Meanwhile the Commanding Officer, with the help of some of the staff, managed to uncouple the burning coaches from the remainder of the train, the patients being transferred to the care of medical officers in an adjacent shed. The next news of the train came from the Railway Transport Officer at Le Mans, who said that what was left of it had passed through bound for La Baule. He also remarked that he could see nothing but heads on board, so many people were there packed on the train. No 4 Ambulance Train eventually reached Rouen.

Another 'happy ending', though incomplete, concerns No 6 Ambulance Train. It was trapped by the advancing front in a little village, after evacuating patients from a Casualty Clearing Station to the base. At about 3 am on 18 May, 1940, an engine joined the train as it stood in its siding. An air raid was in progress and the sky alight with searchlights from Douai, but the train moved on to Albert which was then being evacuated. The first patient to be entrained was a young woman, frightened, distressed and in labour, and accompanied by her mother. She was immediately tended by the nursing sisters, and examination showed that the baby was due to be born by the early evening. But since it was far from safe on the train, the expectant mother and *maman* were taken to a dusty little room behind the platform. Here baby Brigitte was successfully born and at 9.30 pm all three were evacuated in a motor ambulance. No 6 Ambulance Train, however, was not so fortunate. The line was destroyd on either side, and to delay meant to risk being captured. The three nursing sisters were evacuated, but it can only be assumed that the train was to be one of the nine which fell into enemy hands.

There is one more ambulance train story, but the number of the train is unknown. Three days after being at Dieppe, this train had reached Armentières, drawn by an engine crewed by a very old driver and a strapping young girl who acted as a stoker. Outside Armentières the train took on its load of British and Allied wounded. It had accommodation for 340 but as many more as possible were entrained—British, French, Belgian and Indian troop casualties, and also some French children, wounded in their flight from the enemy. By the time daylight came the train had managed to move only a few miles—not only had the track been bombed but there were five refugee trains in front blocking the line. Bombing continued intermittently all morning but by noon had slackened off. There were also some wounded German prisoners on the train, who were apparently completely demoralized by their colleagues' activities. They demanded to be put off the train and taken to a base hospital—a place of relative safety—but it is not known whether their wish was granted. Eventually, however, the train reached a port, and the patients were transferred to a hospital ship, bound for the United Kingdom.

CHAPTER 13

Casualty Evacuation Trains in the United Kingdom in the Second World War

In the Second World War, aircraft development led to the situation wherein Britain herself became part of the fighting line. Thus an essential use of railway ambulance transport at home was expected to be the evacuation and distribution of civilian sick and civilian casualties resulting from air-raids.

In September, 1938, the Ministry of Transport evolved a plan for the evacuation of the London hospitals, and subsequently the Casualty Evacuation Trains Committee was formed. The Chairman was a representative of the Ministry of Transport, with members from the Ministry of Health, the Department of Health for Scotland, the Admiralty, the War Office, the Air Ministry, the Railway Executive Committee and the four main railway companies.

The Committee decided that 21 trains would be required, and that each should be made up of ten parcel and two brake vans; the parcel vans were to be adapted to accommodate approximately 30 stretcher cases each. These plans were made under the threat of war and covered the first emergency clearance of hospitals. But as the political situation eased temporarily the Ministry of Health was able to work out long-term plans for the subsequent transport of casualties.

In March, 1939, the Ministry of Transport was told that in addition to the 21 ambulance trains required for the initial emergency clearance of patients, the Ministry of Health would require additional trains throughout the war, not only in London but also in other large areas of population such as Birmingham, Leeds, Liverpool, Manchester, Newcastle, Sheffield, Southampton and possibly Hull. It was estimated that up to 50

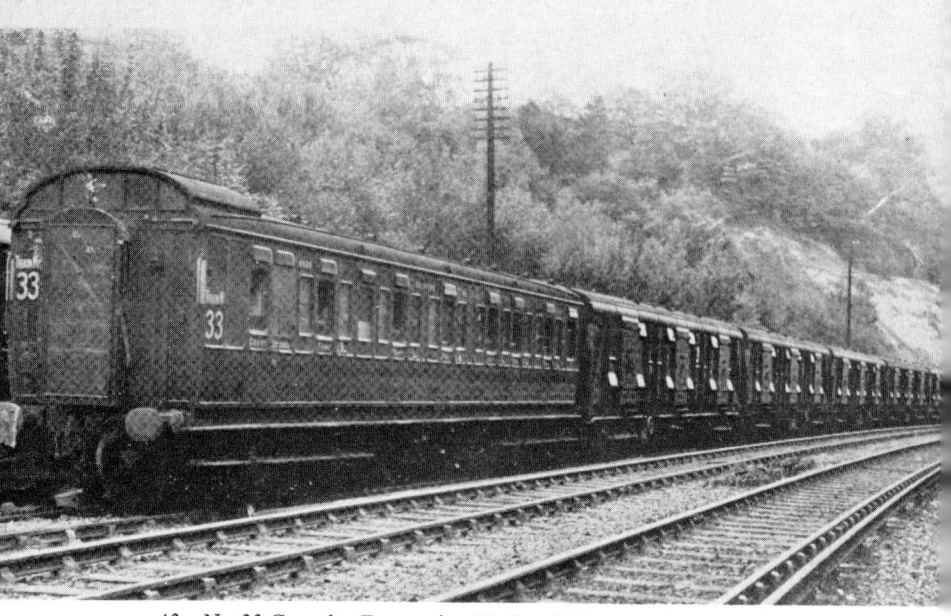

43 No 33 Casualty Evacuation Train which was adapted from Southern Railway rolling stock and used for the evacuation of civilian wounded

trains might be necessary on any one day. On 3 April, however, it was decided that 34 trains would suffice—28 in England, two in Scotland and four on loan to the War Office. By the end of June a prototype van, fitted with brackets for carrying stretchers in two tiers, was accepted. These brackets could easily be removed and carried in containers under the vans. The wagons could then be put into general use, but earmarked for recall for ambulance purposes when necessary.

These improvised ambulance trains were constructed only for the transport of patients who had received treatment and who were fit to travel for comparatively short distances. They were of a much simpler design than the home ambulance trains constructed for troop use by the War Office. They were kept in convenient sidings and their crews billeted nearby, but it was a secret operation of which the public was unaware.

By the end of August, 1939, every civilian hospital in the country had been classified as an 'emergency' hospital. Big mental institutions were cleared of inmates, prefabricated 'hut' hospitals were constructed and casual wards formerly used by vagrants were earmarked for use.

Of the 30 trains reserved for civilians, one was allotted to each of the following towns—Birmingham, Bristol, Exeter, Leeds, Liverpool, Manchester and Newcastle. One went to Scotland and the remaining 22 were distributed around the

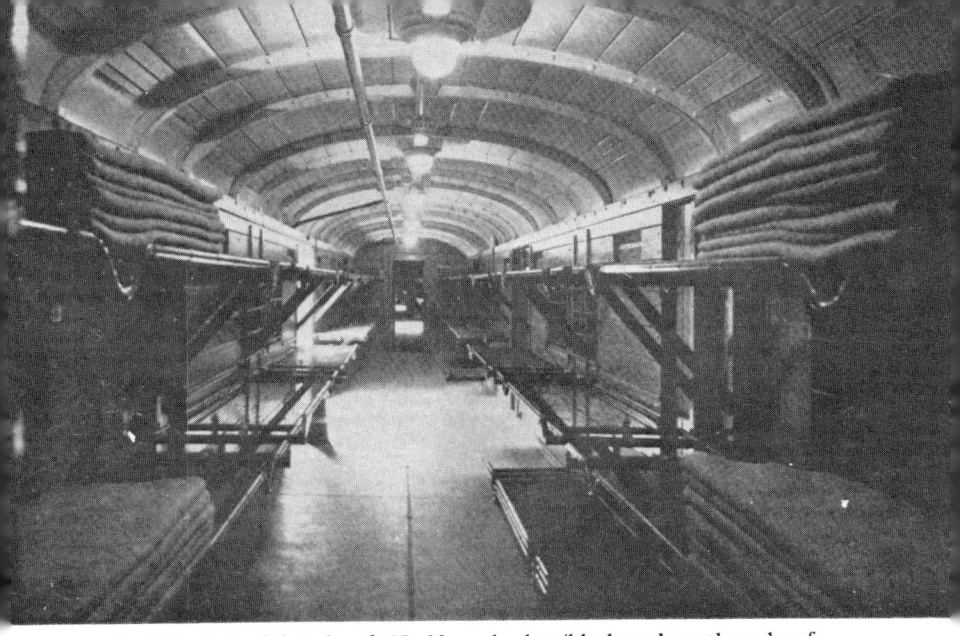

44 The dimly-lit interior of a No 33 coach when 'black-out' was the order of the day

outskirts of London. Most were at their sites by 3 September, and all the London trains had been sited two days later. In October two of the trains which had been loaned to the War Office were returned to the Ministry of Health—one was sent to Scotland and the other was returned to the railway authorities.

The earlier trains, which were composed of assorted rolling stock and three old London and South Western Railway restaurant cars, were converted at the works of the Southern Railway at Lancing and formed into trains in the New Cross yards.

All four railway companies provided some of the Casualty Evacuation Trains, the total of 34 being made up from—Great Western—6; London, Midland and Scottish—15; London and North Eastern—10; Southern –3. Altogether 564 vans and carriages were converted.

These trains were eventually used, as planned, for the clearance of civilian patients from the danger areas, and also for the transport of service sick and wounded from ports of disembarkation, and for transferring large numbers of casualties from one area to another. In carrying service sick and wounded they naturally supplemented the army ambulance trains. Casualty Evacuation Trains were in the end little-used for the transportation of air raid casualties. From the end of May,

1940, to 10 June of that year, apart from civilians, they carried over 28,000 military and nearly 3,500 naval patients.

Casualty evacuation trains were held at five emergency railheads and each railhead had an alternative site. In the early days some were berthed at Tunbridge Wells and subsequently two were held at Sevenoaks. They were manned day and night so as to be available to move emergency cases to the west of England. Other berthing places were Tattenham Corner, Hassocks, Early, Romsey and Bournemouth West.

In December, 1939, because the war had not followed its expected course, and in view of an acute shortage of rolling stock, ten of the 22 trains located near London were disbanded and returned to the railway authorities for general use. They were earmarked for recall when necessary and arrangements made so that they could be re-fitted into ambulance trains and placed in position where required within 72 hours.

In June, 1940, after the collapse of France these ten trains were recalled and the War Office handed back the two which they still held on loan. One was sent to Scotland; at that time there were 30 trains in England and three in Scotland. Later the War Office also released two ambulance trains which had been prepared for overseas and these joined the three in Scotland.

The position was again reviewed in October, 1941, and 14 casualty evacuation trains were released—twelve from England and two from Scotland.

Casualty evacuation trains were made up of twelve vehicles—the marshalling order being one 'brake van third', four stretcher vans; one staff and kitchen car, five stretcher vans and another 'brake van third'.

A 'brake van third' was a third class corridor coach with a guard's van at one end. This was fitted with two water tanks, one of 200 gallons capacity for cold water and the other holding 100 gallons of hot water. Cupboards and shelves were put into two of the compartments for the storage of drugs, dressings and provisions. Another compartment was for the use of the train crew, one was used as an office, another by the Medical Officer, and the last was for the Sister-in-Charge.

The staff and kitchen cars were used as rest rooms for the train crew, as well as for the preparation of meals for patients and staff. The Great Western and Southern Railway Companies provided their own kitchen and dining cars, the kitchen range being removed and replaced by a 'dixie' stove which burnt solid fuel. These stoves had 50 gallon hot water tanks over them.

The London and North Eastern and the London, Midland and Scottish Railways provided a third vestibule van with a guards compartment at the end. This van was fitted as a kitchen with a 'dixie' stove, sinks, cupboards, etc. The seating accommodation of the kitchen cars was: Southern 28; Great Western 30; London and North Eastern 32; London, Midland and Scottish 30.

Stretcher accommodation was provided in bogie vans fitted with removable brackets on which two tiers of stretchers were carried. In addition one row of stretchers could be placed on the floor.

The average train accommodation was 300 stretcher cases, which could be increased to 345 in an emergency.

Stretcher vans were heated by a steam pipe running along the roof and connected to the engine. When not so connected paraffin Aladdin stoves were used. Hurricane lamps and Air Raid Precaution electric torches provided illumination when the train was stationary and there was a louvre ventilator at each end of the van to ensure adequate ventilation when the windows were shut. All windows were blacked-out to conform to Air Raid Precaution Regulations, and they were covered with anti-splinter mesh fabric. The railway companies provided two chemical fire extinguishers to each van, which also carried scoops and sand buckets to deal with incendiary bombs.

The Director-General, Emergency Medical Services, controlled the Casualty Evacuation Trains but their movement was the responsibility of the Railway Executive Committee.

Each train had a staff of a medical officer-in-charge, a hospital train officer who also acted as staff officer, three trained nurses, ten auxiliary nurses and eight orderlies.

The Central Medical War Committee provided the medical officers; the hospital train officers came from the Ministry of Health while the nursing staff were members of the Civil Nursing Reserve. Two superintending sisters supervised the welfare of the nurses, and the orderlies were recruited from the St John Ambulance Brigade. In August, 1940, the hospital train officers were withdrawn and in the same month the senior trained nurse on each train was upgraded to charge sister with responsibility to the medical officer for the staff of the train and also for the equipment.

The original scale of equipment, worked out on the assumption that the patients would probably have received treatment in hospital and would thus require little attention on the journey, was found to be inadequate, and this was increased as supplies became available.

So far as feeding was concerned the original intention was that the patients would bring with them one day's rations (supplied by the discharging hospitals) and this would be supplemented by medical comforts on the train. During the heavy air attacks on the larger cities the discharging hospitals were not always able to provide these rations, and because of this the supplies to the trains were increased, and on the longer journeys a 'knife and fork' meal was given. To enable this to be done three extra auxiliary nurses were added to the train crew. Subsequently much larger stocks of supplies were provided so as to enable each train to cater for its crew and at least 300 patients for a week.

The patients were brought to the train in ambulances or buses, and were loaded on to the train by the train orderlies, being generally carried on metal stretchers. When the patients arrived in a continual stream, about 100 stretcher cases could be loaded in an hour.

The principal movements of the casualty evacuation trains up to the end of 1940 were:—

(a) 1 September, 1939: Initial clearance of London Hospitals
—2,902 patients in 18 trains.

(b) 5 to 11 July, 1940: Clearance of Public Assistance Hospitals on the East Coast—1,727 patients in 9 trains.

(c) 10 September, 1940: Clearance of coastal belt from the Wash to Bournemouth—2,352 patients in 15 trains.

(d) 10 October to 14 November, 1940: Clearance of aged

and infirm from London County Council hospitals—including many homeless from shelters—7,612 patients in 34 trains.

In addition to the above, the casualty evacuation trains cleared reception hospitals during the evacuation from Dunkirk.

The total number of patients carried from D-day to the disbandment of the casualty evacuation train service was 192,551—of whom 152,492 were service cases (101,900 British, 47,319 American and 3,273 Canadian).

Stretcher vans attached to passenger trains also carried 31,186 patients, bringing the total to almost a quarter of a million.

CHAPTER 14

Ambulance Trains and Hospital Ships Today and in the Future

Ambulance Trains

This post-war and present-day history of British Ambulance trains is centred on the British Army of the Rhine (BAOR) where, during 1950–1952, 33 German railway passenger coaches were converted into three ambulance trains, each of 11 vehicles:

    1 kitchen car
    1 pharmacy coach
    1 officers' staff car
    1 other ranks' staff car
    4 ward coaches
    1 compartment ward coach
    2 kitchen wards.

In 1970 these trains were modified and converted for wartime use, the number of vehicles being reduced to nine. The pharmacy coach, the kitchen car and the compartment ward coach were all converted into open ward coaches. One of the kitchen ward coaches was modernized and the other converted to a ward coach with an area for use by a field surgical team if necessary—this being redesignated the 'operating theatre ward'. Thus the wartime make up of the train is:

    1 kitchen car
    1 other ranks' staff coach
    1 officers' staff coach
    1 operating theatre ward
    5 ward coaches.

The ward coaches are fitted with 30 or 36 bed-frames according to the type of the coach—the frames being modified to take stretchers.

Each train has a heater van and a pack wagon while all ward coaches have room for a storage cupboard. Solid fuel heaters have been retained on coaches where originally fitted.

With the addition of a German railway passenger coach, the approximate capacity of each train is for 200 lying and 50 sitting patients.

During the period 1950 to 1953 the trains were used to carry patients from Trieste and Austria to BAOR. They remained in use in BAOR until 1964 when, under what was termed the 'aeromedevac' scheme, the patients were moved by air. During this period they were garaged at Hanover and Rheindahlen and staffed by regular RAMC personnel. In 1964 the trains were handed over to 79 Railway Squadron, Royal Corps of Transport, and the RAMC staff reduced to a cadre—which was ultimately disbanded in 1967.

At the present time the trains are exercised in their war role by RAMC Territorial Army and Voluntary Reserve ambulance train units, who undergo their annual training for two successive years at home and a third year in BAOR. Their 1967 home training was on the Longmoor Military Railway and since then this has been done on 'Ambulance Car—No S 79215' which was purchased from British Railways in 1968, and is garaged at Bramley. (Incidentally this is one of the coaches which has been used for the carriage of Pilgrims to Lourdes.) In 1968, and again in 1971, annual training was carried out in BAOR on one of the actual trains the units would be required to staff should mobilization occur.

The make-up of the 'Ambulance Car' just referred to is much the same as any of the coaches of the old War Department Ambulance Train which was built as long ago as 1900. The official description which refers to it as 'Ambulance Car—army 777' shows that it has three compartments, accommodates 24 lying patients in three tiered cots and has sitting space for 11 other patients. It is fitted with a kitchen with a sink, a water heater, an oven and grill cooker and an ice-box and store. There are the usual toilet and washing facilities and in addition to the general 23 lights there is a bed light over each bunk. The coach is 12 ft 8

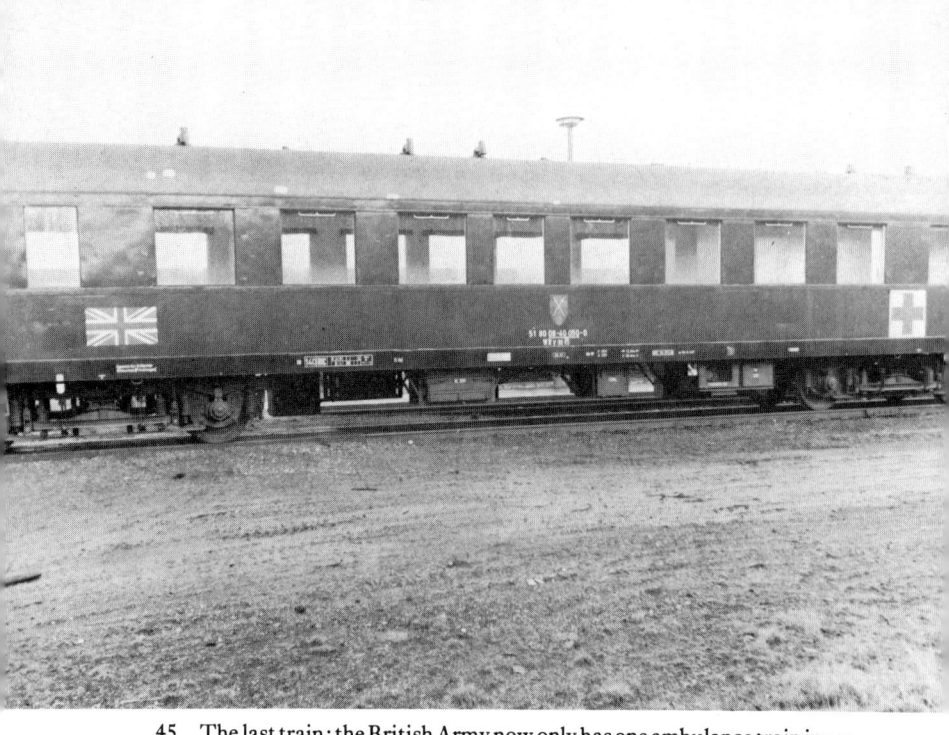

45 The last train: the British Army now only has one ambulance train in service. It is located in BAOR and is used by members of the RAMC (TAVR) when on annual training

ins high, 9 ft wide, 51 ft 7 ins long and has a tare of 32 tons. In addition to the dynamo and battery box it carries propane gas containers.

Military ambulance trains for future use are also similar to the standard type used during the two World Wars. They will have eight ward coaches to accommodate not less than 200 patients, a surgery coach, a kitchen car, separate accommodation coaches for other ranks and officers of the train staff, a heater van, pack wagon and a railway staff van—a total of 15 vehicles. In the ward coaches there is a space for the attendant, who is provided with a table and chair. The gangways will be 3 ft wide and the ambient temperature will be controlled in the range 65° to 70° F. Cooking facilities will provide each patient with one hot meal on his journey, who will also have a water allowance of $2\frac{1}{2}$ gallons for all purposes. Calor gas refrigerators and sterilizers are to be provided; there will be fluorescent strip lighting, and toilet facilities will be of the 'Elsan' closet type. It

158

is understood that consideration is being given to the addition of a special 'operating–theatre' coach which would enable the train to function as a self contained hospital in the event of it being unable to be used in its proper role as an ambulance train.

Hospital ships

It seems that the story of military hospital ships, which in the past have been requisitioned liners taken into use on mobilization, has come to an end. As the normal movement of fit troops for overseas is now done by air and 'troop transports' have ceased to exist, it is reasonable to assume that the movement of all sick and wounded personnel will also be carried out by air in future.

So far as the navy is concerned, it is now without a hospital ship, as HMHS *Maine* was not replaced when she ended her career in 1954. Should one be required in a future emergency, the Royal Yacht *Britannia* is designed to be readily adapted for hospital ship duties.

CHAPTER 15

Appreciation

Through this story there have been a succession of references to the activities of individuals and of Associations, Organizations and Societies who, by voluntary effort, have done so much to help and comfort sick and wounded carried on Ambulance Trains and Hospital Ships.

Once again Florence Nightingale is one of the leaders; in the Crimean War she initiated the issue of gifts and comforts to the British Troops, including scarves knitted by Queen Victoria.

The British Red Cross Society with their never-ending record of voluntary work provided linen, clothing, etc, for a 'hospital' train in the Russo–Turkish War of 1877–1878. Soup and wine were also given to a trainload of wounded at Bucharest in the same war. French bread, rice, soup, medical comforts and warm clothing were provided for the 300 sick and wounded on board the *Osmanieh* during those hostilities.

In the Zulu campaign of 1879 the same Society provided luxuries for patients on homeward-bound transports.

In the Egyptian campaign of 1884–1885 the yacht *Stella* distributed oranges, lemons, limes, bananas, pineapples and other fruits to three hospital ships at Port Said. The Princess of Wales Branch of the National Aid Society also provided comforts to hospital ships in this campaign.

Early in 1900, in the South African War, all sick and wounded carried in hospital trains received a hospital kit contained in a linen bag, on which was stamped in red letters 'The Gift of the Good Hope and British Red Cross Societies'. Each bag held a suit of pyjamas, flannel shirt, a pair of socks, a pair of slippers, handkerchief, towel, tooth-brush, sponge-bag, sponge, hair-brush, and a cake of soap. The recipients called them their 'lucky bags' and their cost—18s each—was borne by the two Societies. By 21 November, 1900, over 14,000 'lucky bags' had been issued when all arrangements for their issue and the cost were taken over by the Good Hope Committee. During the same war the British Red Cross Society supplied comforts to five hospital trains and eight hospital ships.

Similar gift bags—'dorothy-bags'—were given to the sick and wounded by the British Red Cross Society in the First World War. They contained stationery, toilet articles, sweets and cigarettes or tobacco—the bags being of a shape and size to hold a man's small personal belongings as well.

As early as November, 1914, V.A.D.'s gave hot drinks to a small number of walking wounded who had reached Boulogne in an empty supply train, and to some other wounded who were unable to walk and who travelled in trucks on beds of straw.

At Southampton the British Red Cross Society set up a Depot to supply comforts to ambulance trains garaged there and to hospital ships arriving at the port.

One of the first personal voluntary efforts also occurred at Southampton. On the arrival of the earliest Belgian refugees, two sisters, the Misses Tebbut, gave them cigarettes and chocolate. One was a member of the Order of St John of Jerusalem while her sister belonged to the British Red Cross Society. They continued this voluntary aid to the sick and wounded British troops from the arrival of the first hospital ship. They later included postcards, pencils, matches and newspapers among their gifts.

At many of the larger railway stations V.A.D's met ambulance trains and not only gave the patients tea, sandwiches, cake and fruit, but also replenished their supplies of cigarettes, tobacco, matches, post-cards and newspapers.

As a general rule much of the stretcher work at railway stations was carried out by members of voluntary organizations, but on many occasions railway staffs who were trained members of Railway Companies Ambulance Centres helped in the work.

Members of the St Andrew's Ambulance Association and of the British Red Cross Society were much in evidence in the

Glasgow district—removing upwards of 35,000 sick and wounded from ambulance trains arriving there.

In France the British Red Cross Society set up Supply Depots from which were not only eggs, milk, butter and fruit supplied to ambulance trains, but also biscuits, Bengers Food, meat extract, cigarettes, sterilized milk and various items of clothing.

The Society continued its good work in the Second World War. Hospital ships and other vessels received comforts and supplies at Alexandria and Cairo. Red Cross canteens were set up at Suez and at other ports, where patients being transferred from ambulance train to hospital ship were given refreshments. At Tripoli comforts were given to the patients arriving at the docks for embarkation on hospital carriers, while similar issues were made to hospital ships at Syracuse, Tunis and in Italy. The requirements of the hospital carriers during the D-day operations were also met. Another of the amenities provided by the Society was the supply of library books to hospital ships sailing from home ports and to ambulance trains in the United Kingdom.

Lastly, the greatest appreciation is due to the numerous non-service personnel who worked throughout the war, often under the most dangerous and difficult conditions at sea and on land, to the masters and crews of the hospital ships, hospital carriers and ambulance transports for the responsible manner in which they undertook the transport of their convoys of sick and wounded, and to the drivers, firemen, guards and all grades of the staffs of railway companies, at home and abroad, who took such trouble to ensure the efficient running of ambulance trains.

The efforts of all who have been mentioned above and numerous others were of the greatest assistance not only to the patients but also to the medical services of the Forces.

APPENDIX A

Naval Hospital Ships from 1608 to 1731

* Hired merchantman.

Name	Tonnage	Guns	Crew	Dates of Service
Goodwill	—	—	—	1608
Joseph	101	4	30–40	1665
(Loyal) Catherine	298	36–40	35	1665–6
*Maryland Merchant	—	41	40	1666
*Catherine	260	12	40–54	1672–4
*John's Advice	330	16	40–54	1672–4
*Unity	118/120	6–8	—	1683
*Welcome	78	10	—	1683
Helderenberg	242/237	18–30	50	1688
*Concord	352	22–30	45	1690–5
*Society	357	22–30	45	1690–7
*Baltimore	300/324	20	45	1691
*Spencer	245	20	40–45	1691
*London Merchant	250	22–30	30–45	1692–6
*Siam	333	22–30	45–58	1693–7, 1702–3
*Bristol	532	20	40–45	1692–4, 1696–7
Josiah	664	30	30	1696
*Muscovy Merchant	250	24	45	1696
*Princess Anne	484	24–30	70–83	1702–6
*Antelope	550	24–30	60–83	1695, 1702–3 1706–8
*Jeffreys	513	20–26	60	1702–8
Suffold Hagboat	477	8–30	50–70	1701, 1702
Lewis Hulk	460	42	50	1701
Sarah and Betty	370	24	45–58	1702–3
*Smyrna Factor	355	24	45–50	1702–3 1705–9
Suffolk Hoy	–	10–30	80	1703–4
*Matthews	—	—	50–60	1705–8
*Martha	—	22	70–80	1707–10

APPENDIX A

(continued)

Arundel	—	—	—	1709
*Leake	—	14	50–80	1708–11
Pembroke	—	28	60–95	1709–13
Delicia	—	22	63–65	1710–13
Looe	553	12–42	60	1717–18
Portsmouth	—	—	—	1731

APPENDIX B

Hospital Ships on Service with the Royal Navy from 1790 to 1854

Enterprise (off Tower)	1790–1816
Roebuck	1790–1791
Chatham (at Plymouth)	1793–1802
Gladiator (at Portsmouth)	1793–1802
Grana	1793–1800
Le Caton (at Plymouth)	1794–1798
Le Pegase (at Portsmouth)	1794–1809
Sultan (at Portsmouth)	1794–1796
L'Engageante (at Cork)	1795–1801
Spanker	1796–1802
Argonaut	1797–1828
Africa	1798–1800
Antgalican	1800–1801
Courser	1800
Standard	1800
Matilda	1800–1806
Prince Frederick	1800–1804
Sussex	1801–1816
Trent	1803–1816
Tromp	1803–1810
Wilhelmina (Prince of Wales Island)	1803–1812
Princess	1807 1816
Gorgon	1808–1814
Batavia	1809–1817
Triton	1810–1813
Minden	1842–1846
Alligator	1847–1848
Belle Isle	1854
Union	1793–1802 and 1837

Hospital Muster Books. PRO ADM 102/1.

165

APPENDIX C

Military Hospital Ships and Ambulance Transports in the First World War

Name	Period of Service From To	Accommodation	Remarks
St Andrew	19. 8.14–29. 5.19	194	
St David	19. 8.14–16. 1.19	194	
St Patrick	19. 8.14–26. 1.19	191	
Devanah	22. 8.14–28. 2.19	524	
Asturius	28. 8.14.–21. 3.17	896	T. 21. 3.17
Carisbrook Castle	3. 9.14–26. 8.19	439	
Glengorm Castle	10. 9.14– ***	423	
Sicilia	10. 9.14–11. 9.18	336	
Oxfordshire	15. 9.14–24. 3.18	562	
Guildford Castle	22. 9.14–19.11.18	427	T. 10. 3.18
Gloucester Castle	24. 9.14– 9. 9.19	410	T. 30. 3.17
Glenart Castle	30. 9.14–26. 2.18	453	M. 1. 3.17 & 26. 2.18
Loyalty	2.10.14–30.11.18	325	
Madras	2.10.14– 4.11.19	450*	
Syria	2.10.14–10. 2.20	397	
Varsova	8.10.14– 8. 5.20	475*	
St Dennis	12.10.14–18.10.19	231	
Goorkha	20.10.14–18.10.17	408	M. 10.10.17
Letitia	18.11.14– 1. 8.17	549	
Gascon	25.11.14–15. 2.20	434	
Valdivia	29.11.14–22.12.19	551	
Salta	3.12.14– 9. 4.17	461	M. 10. 4.17
Nevasa	8. 1.15–25. 3.18	660	
Delta	14. 1.15–19. 3.18	530	
Brighton	18. 3.15–15. 5.20	140	
Anglia	25. 4.15–17.11.15	275	M. 17.11.15
Dieppe	6. 5.15– 7. 4.17	167	
Newhaven	7. 5.15– 5. 3.19	163	

Name	Period of Service From To	Accommodation	Remarks
St. George	7. 5.15– 4.12.17	278	
Massilia	12. 5.15–25. 3.16	375	
Assaye	16. 5.15– 2. 3.20	488	
Maheno	25. 5.15– 2. 6.19	515	
Dongola	25. 5.15–11. 7.19	506	
Neuralia	12. 6.15–31. 7.19	630	
Grantully Castle	22. 6.15–11. 3.19	552	
Galeka	22. 6.15–28.10.16	366	M. 28.10.16
Formosa	23. 6.15– 7. 7.19	417	
Dunluce Castle	6. 7.15– 2. 4.19	755	
Panama	25. 7.15–23.11.19	484	
Egypt	2. 8.15– 1. 6.19	461	
Cambria	8. 8.15–20. 1.19	189	
Takada	10. 8.15–29. 4.19	450*	
Dover Castle	11. 8.15–26. 5.17	607	T. 26. 5.17
Karoola	11. 8.15– 6.11.18	523	
Ebani	13. 8.15–12.10.19	508	
Tagus	24. 8.15–31. 3.16	418	
Kanowna	26. 8.15– 8. 7.19	424	
Karapara	27. 8.15–20. 2.16	341	
Jan Breydel	27. 8.15– 1. 8.19	158	
Essequibo	2. 9.15–12. 9.19	589	
Aquitania	4. 9.15–27.12.17	4,182	
Varela	2.10.15– ***	450*	
Stad Antwerpen	2.10.15–12.12.19	165	
Dunvegan Castle	6.10.15–20. 4.16	400	
Kildonan Castle	6.10.15–10. 3.16	603	
Lanfranc	6.10.15–17. 4.17	403	T. 17. 4.17
Braemar Castle	7.10.15– 1. 8.19	421	M. 23.11.16
Morea	8.10.15–28. 3.16	750	
Aberdonian	16.10.15–16. 6.19	245	
Western Australia	21.10.15– 6.12.18	305	
Mauretania	22.10.15– 1. 3.16	1,945	
Vita	27.10.15–24. 2.20	405*	
Ellora	12.11.15–10. 1.20	475*	
Britannic	13.11.15–21.11.16	3,310	M. 21.11.16
Copenhagen	1. 1.16– 5. 3.17	254	
Erinpura	1. 5.16–13. 6.19	475*	
Herefordshire	25. 7.16– 1. 1.18	380	
Warilda	25. 7.16– 3. 8.18	546	T. 3. 8.18
Llandovery Castle	26. 7.16–27. 6.18	622	T. 27. 6.18
Wandilla	5. 8.16–15. 3.18	549	
Princess Elizabeth	8.11.16– 3. 9.19	30	

Name	Period of Service		Accommodation	Remarks
	From	To		
Marama	Period doubtful		97	
Pieter de Connick	16. 3.17–28. 3.19		377	
Araguaya	2. 5.17– 8.11.19		840	
Kalyan	4. 5.17–29.11.19		821	
Vasna	29. 5.17– ***		613	
Ville de Liege	13. 6.17–30.12.18		173	
Donegal	No details available			T. 17. 4.17

The following yachts were also employed for carrying sick and wounded.

Sheelah	Gift	August, 1914	– February, 1919
Albion	Gift	30 October, 1914	– about 21 February, 1915
Queen Alexandra	Gift	February, 1915	– about 20 January, 1919
Grianaig	Gift	4 July, 1918	– about February, 1919

Prince George — Requisitioned by the Canadian Government and released almost immediately.

Notes

***	Still in service in 1921
*	Approximate accommodation
M.	Mined
T.	Torpedoed

Figures given for the *Delta* are for it as a hospital carrier, no other figures being available.

APPENDIX D

Hospital Ships and Other Vessels used for the Reception, Treatment and Movement of Casualties During the Gallipoli Campaign of 1915/1916

Hospital ships and carriers

Aquitania
Braemar Castle
Britannic
Delta
Devanah
Dongola
Dunluce Castle
Galeka
Gascon
Gloucester Castle
Goorkha
Grantala (Australian Naval Hospital Ship)
Guildford Castle
Karanowna (Australian)
Karoola (Australian)
Letitia
Maheno (New Zealand)
Mauretania
Neuralia
Sicilia
Somali (Royal Navy)
Soudan (Royal Navy)

Transports, troopships and other vessels

Alauria
Aragon
Arcadian
Ascarius
Caledonian
Clan MacGillivray
Dufflinger
Franconia
Georgia
Hindoo
Ionian
Itonus

Kyarra
Liberty (Yacht)
Lutzow
Mashobra
Osmanieh
Seang Bee
Seang Choon
Southland

APPENDIX E

Naval and Military Hospital Ships and Carriers in the Second World War

Indenta-tion No.	Name	Invalid accommoda-tion	Medical staff	Crew	Remarks
34	Aba	450/484	83	121	
7	Amarapoora	503	103	153	
41	Amra	475	101	177	
64	Amsterdam	*	*	*	Sunk August, 1944
33	Atlantis	623	97	200	
50	Batavier II	216	51	55	
31	Brighton	*	*	*	Bombed and sunk 21 May, 1940
*	Bury	*	*	*	
57	Cap St Jacques	432	88	160	
63	Chantilly	611	96	159	
28	Dinard	221	59	79	Mined but reached port.
23	Dorsetshire	493	92	168	Bombed–1941
65	Duke of Argyll	416	60	100	
56	Duke of Lancaster	408	60	100	
62	Duke of Rothesay	393	58	100	
53	El Nil	451	85	132	
54	Empire Clyde	426	86	185	
67	Gerusalemme	388/450	*	*	
*	Gripsholm	*	*	*	
26	Isle of Guernsey	*	*	*	
3	Isle of Jersey	160	59	69	
36	Karapara	388	123	182	
60	Karoa	411	89	197	
55	Lady Connaught	335	62	74	
56	Lady Nelson	514	91	114	
37	Leinster	389	63	99	
66	Letitia	758	198	210	
39	Llandovery Castle	450	86	139	
21	Maid of Kent	*	*	*	Bombed and sunk 21 May, 1940
1	Maine	*	*	*	
40	Manunda	327	120	114	
42	Maunganui	364	112	118	
D6	Melchior Treub	300	87	112	
*	Melrose Abbey	*	*	*	
49	Naushon	300	59	66	
38	Newfoundland	*	*	*	Bombed and sunk off Salerno 13 September, 1943
D4	Ophir	332/346	84	215	
D1	Oranje	791	129	277	
6	Oxfordshire	500	98	127	

Indentation No.	Name	Invalid accommodation	Medical staff	Crew	Remarks
32	Paris	*	*	*	Bombed and sunk 2 June 1940
52	Perak	141	35	70	
61	Prague	429	56	103	
58	Principessa Giovanna	402	70	136	
*	RAMB IV	*	*	*	
	Roebuck	*	*	*	Mined but reached port
24	St Andrew	267	58	93	
27	St David	*	*	*	Sunk–25 January 1944
*	St Helier	*	*	*	
29	St Julien	219	59	72	
25	Somersetshire	507	118	171	Torpedoed–April 1942
*	Stockport	*	*	*	? Torpedoed–23 February 1943
35	Tairea	506	120	175	
43	Talamba	485	*	*	Bombed and sunk off Sicily.
D3	Tjitjalengka	504/520	111	135	
59	Toscana	567	88	174	
4	Vasna	279	73	129	
8	Vita	240	76	168	
45	Wanganella	434	102	123	
30	Worthing	*	*	*	
44	Wu Sueh	296	95	65	

* Details not available.

APPENDIX F

Admissions of Patients to Naval Hospital Ships during the Second World War

Hospital ship	1939	1940	1941	1942	1943	1944	1945	Total
Amarapoora	58	3,063	2,746	2,479	212	615	594	9,767
Cap St Jacques	—	—	—	—	—	—	1,207	1,207
Empire Clyde	—	—	—	—	—	—	237	237
Gerusalemme	—	—	—	—	—	—	464	464
Isle of Jersey	—		868	1,529	2,511	2,646	1,739	851	10,144
Maine	168	626	1,764	1,405	5,459	2,276	1,816	13,514
Ophir	—	—	—	—	1,035	7,034	4,042	12,111
Oxfordshire	160	1,961	2,111	1,102	7,753	7,304	1,940	22,331
Tjitjalengka	—	—	—	668	1,599	3,456	1,547	7,270
Vasna	—	890	1,877	1,532	1,872	4,591	1,650	12,412
Vita	—	*	*	1,304	401	592	1,388	3,685
							Total	93,142

* Numbers not recorded.

APPENDIX G

The 'Princess Christian Hospital Train' in the South African War

This train was specially constructed in England for use with the troops in the South African War. It was made up of seven bogie corridor coaches each about 36 ft long and 8 ft wide with a 2 ft 6 ins continuous passage running through the centre. With a total length of 250 ft it accommodated 74 lying patients and its staff. It was painted white for identification purposes and when the coaches arrived from England the train was assembled at Durban in February, 1900.

The first coach was divided into three compartments, one for two nurses, one for two invalid officers and the third for linen and stores.

The next coach was similarly divided, the first compartment for two medical officers and the others for use as a dispensary and dining room respectively.

The four ward coaches each accommodated eighteen patients and four orderlies. The beds which were in three tiers were so arranged that they could be lifted out of the coaches. They were fitted with cupboards and drawers for linen, clothing, medical and surgical supplies, crockery, cutlery, glass and provisions. There were two lockers in the roof also for linen. Each ward coach had a stove and washing and toilet facilities.

The last coach was a kitchen with berths for two cooks and also a compartment for the guard.

There were large cisterns for cold water storage and two large filters and a refrigerator on the train.

It had enamelled white ironwork and fittings and bright draperies and was light and airy. To shelter invalids who were exposed to the sun when they were being entrained there was an awning suspended from hooks over the carriage doors supported by telescopic iron posts.

In the centre panel on the outside of each coach was a Red Cross on a white background encircled by the words 'Princess Christian Hospital Train'. It carried the Union Jack and the Red Cross in sockets at the head displayed in accordance with Article VII of the Geneva Convention of 22 August, 1864.

APPENDIX H

No. 4 Hospital Train in the South African War

This was an improvised train made up in South Africa, with a dining-car and a kitchen which had belonged to the Orange Free State Railway forming the nucleus. To this was added a post office van and a bogie truck which had already been converted for hospital train purposes with iron frames and springs sent out from England at the beginning of the war and which had been used on the Eastern line in charge of an NCO of the Cape Medical Staff Corps. A third class coach, a second class saloon and another kitchen were added. The result was a five coach train which was taken into use on 10 June, 1900. In the first coach were separate compartments for two medical officers and two nursing sisters. The next was a kitchen car with a range, a meat safe and store cupboards; this portion was shut off by doors from two mess rooms and sleeping accommodation for seven NCOs and orderlies. The third coach was for patients and reserved as far as possible for cases of enteric fever. The fourth accommodated surgical patients and the other was the officers' ward. Later two more coaches were added making a total accommodation for 114 patients including six officers in their own compartment. Still later two small vans were attached for kits, pack-store and the guard.

The beds of this train consisted of moveable iron brackets with sheet canvas and hair mattresses, sheets, blankets and coloured counterpanes. They were so constructed that they could be folded up and so allow space for chairs for sitting cases. There was a continuous passage through the train and each coach had its own toilet facilities. Water was carried underneath the vehicles and each ward coach had folding doors on each side to allow the easy entrainment of patients on stretchers.

The interior was painted green and the outside painted white and was often referred to as the 'White Train'. Each coach had the number of the train and a Red Cross painted on the outside.

APPENDIX J

Growth of the Military Ambulance Train Service in France in the First World War

Train number	Date of entry into service		Railway providing rolling stock	Accommodation Lying	Sitting
1	1914 August	24	Etat	308	17
2		25	Etat and PLM	228	154
3		26	Etat and PLM	233	98
4		30	Nord	354	—
6	Sept	5	Nord	272	— (a)
5		16	Etat and PLM	212	224
7		20	Etat and PLM	260	41
8	Oct	8	Etat and Nord	231	84
9		31	Etat and PLM	271	28
12	Nov	12	GE & LNW	280	— (b)
10		13	Etat	280	180
11	Dec	15	Etat	262	— (c)
16	1915 April	24	GW	162	320 (d)
17		25	GE	160	280 (d)
14	May	26	LBSC & LNW	158	280 (e)
15	June	1	B'ham R & CW Co	264	116 (f)
22	August	20	LNW	162	280
21		25	LNW	162	280
24	Sept	17	L & Y	162	320
18		27	GW	162	320
20	1916 Jan	5	GE	162	280
19	Feb	8	GW	192	266
23	March	3	Caledonian	162	292
25		25	LB & SC	162	329
29	April	26	L & Y	306	64
26	May	14	GW	306	64
30		27	L & NW	306	56
31	June	16	L & NW	306	56
27		24	GW	306	64
28	July	10	GE	306	56

Train number	Date of entry into service	Railway providing rolling stock		Accommodation Lying	Sitting
38	1917 July	21	London	302	33
36	August	12	GE	306	72
33		28	GW	306	80
32	Sept	2	L & NW	306	72
34		28	Midland	306	80
37	Nov	25	NE	306	72
41	Dec	12	L & NW	356	39
35		20	L & SW	306	80
42	1918 Jan	16	L & Y	356	39
39		28	GW	356	39
43	June	3	GW	356	39

Notes — (a) Franco-British Train
       (b) Khaki Train
       (c) Provided by the British Red Cross Society
       (d) Provided by the United Kingdom Flour Millers Association
       (e) Queen Mary's Ambulance Train
       (f) Princess Christian Hospital Train

APPENDIX K

Capacity of Military Ambulance Trains in France, September, 1915

Designation	With maximum lying patients			With maximum sitting patients		
	Lying	Sitting	Total	Lying	Sitting	Total
No 1	188	77	265	88	461	549
2	184	182	366	—	561	561
3	215	20	235	135	340	475
4	227	74	301	160	267	427
5	130	133	263	48	298	346
6	144	72	216	35	513	548
7	176	134	310	94	401	495
8	235	90	325	111	600	711
9	144	188	332	72	466	538
10	158	284	442	92	516	608
11	234	—	234	—	410	410
12	220	40	260	—	370	370
14	144	256	400	48	448	496
15	174	220	394	58	458	516
16	152	320	472	48	532	580
17	120	210	330	120	280	400

APPENDIX L

First Battle of the Somme. Evacuation of casualties by Ambulance Train from 1 to 4 July, 1916

Table I Train journeys and numbers of patients carried

Date		Ambulance train	Temporary ambulance train	Journeys	Total Patients
1 July	Journeys	5	—	5	
	Patients	2,317	—		2,317
2 July	Journeys	14	4	18	
	Patients	7,661	3,638		11,299
3 July	Journeys	17	6	23	
	Patients	8,492	4,894		13,386
4 July	Journeys	14	3	17	
	Patients	4,239	2,151		6,390
Totals	Journeys	50	13	63	
	Patients	22,709	10,683		33,392*

* includes over 1,000 officers

Table II Railheads and bases

Railheads.	Patients entrained	Bases	Patients detrained
Doullens	811	Boulogne	5,720
Gezaincourt	8,610	Étaples	4,178
Heilly	6,225	Havre	1,006
Puchevillers	4,658	Le Tréport	340
Vequement	12,095	Rouen	18,328
Unspecified	993	Unspecified	3,820
Total	33,392	Total	33,392

Table III Details of ambulance and temporary ambulance trains—showing numbers of patients carried.

Ambulance train number	Authorised accommodation	1 July	2 July	3 July	4 July	Total
3	331	445	—	—	—	445
4	354	—	—	—	107	107
6	272	—	786	417	393	1,596
7	301	—	624	541	—	1,165
8	315	449	—	—	—	449
9	299	—	—	400	397	797
10	460	—	641	449	149	1,239
11	262	—	543	625–607*	297	2,072
12	280	—	—	—	318	318
15	380	516	462	296	335	1,609
16	482	—	—	386	—	386
18	482	420	380	586	374	1,760
19	458	—	439	400	—	839
20	442	487	474	309	212	1,482
21	442	—	—	563	226	789
22	442	—	531	556	273	1,360
24	482	—	589	—	—	589
25	491	—	515	—	214–523*	1,252
29	370	—	761	621	—	1,382
30	362	—	579	408	421	1,408
31	362	—	337	871–457*	—	1,665
	Totals	2,317	7,661	8,492	4,239	22,709

Temporary Ambulance Trains. Number

		1 July	2 July	3 July	4 July	Total
102		—	993	340	—	1,333
104		—	999	1,006	—	2,005
106		—	863	834	—	1,697
108		—	783	—	—	783
110		—	—	1,053	718	1,771
114		—	—	614	969	1,583
116		—	—	1,047	—	1,047
118		—	—	—	464	464
	Totals	—	3,638	4,894	2,151	10,683

Total number of patients carried:

1 July	2,317
2 July	11,299
3 July	13,386
4 July	6,390
Whole period	33,392

* Two journeys on one day

APPENDIX M

Description of No. 63 American Ambulance Train for service in France in the First World War

Medical designation	Description	Accommodation
A 10	Brake van with 4 infectious wards.	1 guard 24 lying infectious cases.
B	Staff car.	3 medical officers 3 nurses.
D 1	Kitchen car with sitting room for officers.	3 cooks 10 officers.
A 1 A 2 A 3 A 4	Ward cars each of 36 berths.	144 lying cases
F	Pharmacy car.	12 serious lying cases.
A 5 A 6 A 7 A 8 A 9	Ward cars each of 36 berths.	180 lying cases.
D 2	Kitchen car with mess room.	2 N.C.O's
C	Personnel car.	33 orderlies.
E	Brake and stores car.	1 guard.

This train was constructed at the Dukinfield works by the Great Central Railway, the 16 coaches having an exterior finish of khaki and each prominently lettered US and embellished with the Red Cross on each side.

With the exception of the brake compartments at each end it was vestibuled throughout and the interior enamelled white. It carried 3,149 gallons of water, was equipped with electric lighting and had both fixed and portable electric fans. In addition to the Westinghouse brakes there was a screw hand brake on each vehicle to accord with American practice.

APPENDIX N

Description of standard Ambulance Trains for Service Overseas in the First World War

These trains had sixteen coaches lettered S, G, A, B, C, D, E, F, L, M, N, O, P, H, R and T, which was the sequence in which the train was marshalled.

Coach S was a brake van and infectious ward and was divided into six sections—one 5 ft long for the guard and one 10 ft long for his living accommodation; another was for the attendants and stretchers whilst the other three sections each accommodated six lying cases.

Coach G was the staff car and this had nine separate sections—three with sleeping, dining and toilet facilities for the nursing sisters; the remaining sections slept the medical officers and contained their mess room and a toilet. The mess room had a dining table, chairs, cupboards and shelves with a seat capable of being used as a bed. This car had a stove and its own hot water system for use when the train was standing in sidings. There was a shower at each end of the coach.

Coach A served a dual purpose being a kitchen car with room for sick officers and sleeping accommodation for three cooks plus a toilet. The kitchen section had a standard army range with a copper boiler with recesses in the hot plate for the boiling pans. It had a dresser, washing up sink and its own supply of hot and cold water. The cold water tanks were in the roof; they held 300 gallons and were fitted with gauges. Similar tanks were fitted in all other coaches.

Coaches B, C, D, and E were ward cars each with thirty-six beds arranged in three tiers, eighteen on either side; they had toilet and washing facilities at the end.

Coach F, the pharmacy car, was divided into five sections: one for the pharmacy itself and separate sections for the treatment room and office and two store rooms. The pharmacy, which had its own water supply, had a hot water heater, a sink, cupboards and shelves. It was immediately adjacent to the treatment room in which there was a portable operating table and a sterilizing tank. The door to the treatment room had a clear opening of 8 ft enabling stretchers to be carried in direct from outside the train. In addition to tables, chairs and a cupboard there was a safe in the office section.

Coaches L, M, N and O were also thirty-six bedded ward cars constructed to the same pattern as the others.

Coach P was an ordinary corridor coach of seven or eight compartments which was devoid of upholstery and could hold 56 sitting cases; it had an upper berth above each seat for 'bad' sitting patients. There were toilet facilities at one end and a pantry at the other.

Coach H was the second kitchen fitted up similarly to coach A; it was also the mess car for both NCOs and privates.

Coach R was the sleeping compartment for the other ranks of the staff; it was similar to a ward car except that shelves for packs, equipment, etc. replaced the upper tier of the beds. It also had its own self-contained heating apparatus.

Coach T was a second brake van and store car of five sections; two for stores, one which included a meat safe for supplies; one for the guard when the train was in motion and the other as his living room.

The trains were 950 ft long and weighed 450 tons. They came into service in France in 1916.

APPENDIX O

Miltiary Ambulance Trains in the United Kingdom in the First World War

Outbreak of war

Home ambulance trains, which were numbered consecutively, were made up to a standard pattern of nine vehicles from corridor coaches, parcel vans, dining cars and brake vans; they were about 350 ft long and weighed 250 tons.

There were five ward coaches with beds in two tiers and each could accommodate twenty lying cases; when the upper berths were loaded they could take thirty 'sitters'. There was a pharmacy car which included a treatment room, office and store accommodation. The kitchen car had a pantry and dining space for sitting patients and beds for some of the other rank staff. Another coach had berths for two medical officers, two nursing sisters and two other ranks, while six more of the other ranks slept in the ninth coach which had store accommodation and room for the guard.

Two ordinary corridor passenger coaches for the use of sitting patients and another kitchen car were subsequently added.

The establishment of these trains was 1 medical officer, 2 nursing sisters and 12 other ranks. Cooks were occasionally provided by the railway company which fitted out the train.

New standard type

This was made up of ten vehicles, the first with separate accommodation for the guard, two medical officers and two nurses; next was a combined dining and sleeping car which accommodated six orderlies; then came six ward cars each with beds for twenty patients; there was also a pharmacy and office car while the last vehicle was for the use of the remaining orderlies, the carriage of stores and accommodation of the guard. These trains were 350 feet long and weighed 250 tons and had self-contained heating apparatus for use when heat was not provided by the engines; a Geneva Cross in ten inch red and white squares was painted on both sides of all coaches. When extra accommodation was needed bogie vans which each carried twenty patients on stretchers or passenger coaches for 'sitters' were attached.

APPENDIX P

Description of the War Department Ambulance Train – the 'Netley Coaches'

This train was made up of five identical coaches each 48 ft long and just over 8 ft wide outside. Each coach was divided into three compartments the first being 8 ft long and used either for an invalid or a medical officer. It had two first class seats capable of being converted into a bed. Partitioned off was a lavatory and there were also two cupboards, some racks and a linen chest.

The central and main compartment was 31 ft 3 ins long with entrance doorways 4 ft wide on either side. It contained 12 Fieldhouse patent spring beds in two tiers and had two seats which each took three sitting patients. The beds were so constructed that they could be lifted off their fittings.

Another 8 ft long compartment was at the other end of the ward and it seated three patients; it had a partitioned lavatory and a space contained an oil gas stove for the preparation of hot drinks; there was a rack for cooking utensils.

The interior of the coach, with the exception of the mahogany fittings of the seats and doors, was white enamelled; the upholstery was dark maroon leather and the floor was covered with corticine. Each coach had 26 side ventilators with moveable shutters and 14 torpedo air extractors on the roof; there were 16 drop lights and 6 large and 2 small lamps worked on the Pintsch's system of gas lighting. This was subsequently replaced by electric light supplied by dynamos. Each coach had its own hot water system.

The train was built on the central corridor principle with sliding doors at each end gangway which enabled the coaches to be used individually; it was fitted with Westinghouse air-pressure brakes.

The exterior was distinctively painted with French grey top panels and khaki on the lower panels and fascias, the latter being picked out with yellow and fine-lined with red. There were two Geneva Crosses on each side of each coach with the Royal Arms emblazoned on one of the French grey panels. 'War Department Ambulance Coach' was painted on the lower portion of each coach side. A sixth coach was subsequently added.

APPENDIX Q

No. 1 Naval Ambulance Train in the United Kingdom in the First World War

This was a unit of the Medical Transport system organised by the Nore Command and consisted of twelve London and North Western corridor vehicles. The make-up of the train was—guards van; seven compartment corridor coach; two cot coaches; a day coach; three cot coaches; store coach; kitchen car with dining saloon; family saloon; rear guards van. The overall buffer to buffer length was 568 feet.

The front guards van in addition to being used by the guard accommodated sixteen of the train crew in hammocks.

The seven-compartment corridor coach was for sitting patients, six being allotted to each compartment.

The five cot coaches were converted parcels vans—45 ft long, 7 ft high at the sides rising to 8 ft in the centre by means of a clerestory. Two sliding doors at the ends gave access to adjoining coaches and there were two 4 ft 6 ins sliding doors on each side which were equidistant from each end of the coach. They were steam-heated by overhead pipes in the clerestory and illuminated by incandescent gas lamps. Four of these coaches each took twenty-four ratings in cots. The other was used by officers and when circumstances allowed the cots were suspended by lanyards in the centre. Washable canvas screens were fitted to the doors and individual cots could be screened off when necessary.

The 'day' coach was a converted parcels van similar to the cot coaches. At one end were two w.c.'s; at the other there were two padded rooms 6 ft by 3 ft 7 ins on one side and a small dressing station on the other. On each side of the central portion of the coach were eight wash basins fitted with a water supply; when not in use they could be covered by a flap hinged to the side of the coach and serve as a table for meals or similar purposes. Collapsible forms enabled twenty-eight patients to take meals at one sitting.

The kitchen car or 'galley' provided meals for the patients and staff.

The family saloon had three compartments, the ends having berths for two medical officers and two nursing sisters respectively, the centre compartment being a sitting room.

The store coach, technically known in railway circles as a 'brake–third', had five ordinary compartments and the guards van. It had lockers for clean and soiled linen and bedding, racks for ward utensils and a safe for valuables. One of the compartments was used for dry stores and groceries, another as an office and a third for the cook and senior sick berth steward. The others were for use as isolation cabins or for other purposes.

The normal accommodation of the train was 120 cot and 72 sitting cases. There was also sitting space for ten officer patients in the dining room and eight could be slept in cots specially made to fit across seats in the saloon. Additional seating for ratings was available in the brake vans which carried folding seats for this purpose.

The maximum number of patients carried on No 1 Naval Ambulance Train on any trip up to 31 December, 1914, was 363. Up to that date the train had made 14 trips, travelled 8,841 miles and carried 1,759 patients of whom 536 were cot cases; the total number of patients was made up of Royal Navy 799, Army 497, Belgians 428 and Germans 35.

BIBLIOGRAPHY

1868 *A Treatise on the Transport of Sick and Wounded Troops*, Deputy-Inspector-General T. Longmore.
1887 *Nor'ard of the Dogger*, E. J. Mather.
1893 *A Manual of Ambulance Transport*, Surgeon-General Sir T. Longmore.
Manual of the Medical Staff Corps.
1899 *The Royal Navy. A History.* Sir W. Laird Clowes.
1902 *Report by the Central Red Cross Committee on Voluntary Organization in aid of Sick and Wounded during the South African War.*
1904 *Medical Arrangements in the South African War*, Sir W. D. Wilson, HMSO.
1904 *Toilers of the Deep.*
1906 *History of the War in South Africa—1899–1902*, General Sir F. Maurice.
1909 *'Times' History of the South African War.*
1911 *The Life and Letters of Sir John Hall*, S. M. Mitra.
Royal Army Medical Corps Training Manual.
North Sea Fishers and Fighters.
1914 *Monthly Army List—August*, HMSO.
Royal Army Medical Corps Seniority Roll of W.O.'s and N.C.O.'s.
1915 *'The Princess Christian Hospital Train'*, British Medical Journal.
Medical Arrangements of the BEF, British Medical Journal.
A Simple Method of Transporting Cot Cases by Ambulance Train, Elder Surgeon A. Vavasour. RNVR. Journal of the Royal Naval Medical Service.

Notes on Ambulance Trains and description of Naval Ambulance Train No 1. Elder Surgeon A. Vavasour. RNVR. Journal of the Royal Naval Medical Service.
The Rise of Rail Power in War and Conflict, E. A. Pratt.
Diary of a Nursing Sister on the Western Front—1914–1915, K. E. Luard, RRC.
1916 *War on the Line*, Bernard Darwin.
British and Continental Ambulance Trains. Lancashire and Yorkshire Railway, F. E. Gobey (a lecture).
Exhibition of a Lancashire and Yorkshire Ambulance Train, John F. Aspinal.
1917 *Roll of Commissioned Officers in the Medical Service of the British Army*, Colonel William Johnston, CB. Aberdeen University Press.
Ambulance Light Trollies, British Medical Journal.
The story of British VAD work in the Great War, Thelka Bowser.
British Medicine in the War—1914–1917, British Medical Journal.
1918 *Southampton Pictorial War Album, 1914–1918*.
The Fitting out and Administration of a Hospital Ship, Flag-Surgeon E. Sutton.
1919 *Lines of Communication* (a souvenir volume), Friends Ambulance Unit, No 17 Ambulance Train, BEF France.
1919 *War Diaries—No 39 Ambulance Train, PRO*.
1920 *Improvised Ambulance Train*, Major R. W. D. Leslie, Journal of the Royal Army Medical Corps.
1921 *Birth and Early days of Ambulance Trains in France—1914–1915*, Major G. A. Moore ('Wagon Lit'), Journal of the Royal Army Medical Corps.
Official History of the War, Committee of Imperial Defence.
British Railways in the Great War, Edwin A. Pratt.
Report of the Joint War Committee of the British Red Cross Society/Order of St John of Jerusalem, 1914–1919.
1922 *The Birth and Early Days of Our Ambulance Trains in France—August 1914*, Colonel G. A. Moore ('Wagon Lit').
Statistics of the Military Effort of the British Empire—1914–1920, HMSO.
1923 *Official History of the 1914–1918 War—Medical Services*, HMSO.
1929 *A Short History of the Royal Army Medical Corps*, Colonel Fred Smith.
1930 *Unknown Warriors*, Sister K. E. Luard, RRC.
The Australian Medical Service of the War, 1914–1918, Australian War Memorial.
1934 *Early Victorian England—Vol 2*, Humphrey Milford.
1936 *A History of the Southern Railway*, C. F. Dendy Marshall.
The Mariner's Mirror—Vol 22.
1937 *The Army Medical Services in War*, Lieut-Colonel T. B. Nicholls.
The Mariners Mirror—Vol. 23.

1939 *Ambulance Handbook of the St Andrew's Ambulance Association.*
Sea Transport Services—Regulations and Instructions, HMSO.
Monthly Army List—September, HMSO.
1940 *The Organisation and Running of an Ambulance Train*, Major C. C. H. Chavasse, Journal of the Royal Army Medical Corps.
1944 *My Early Life*, The Rt Hon Winston S. Churchill.
1945 *The Royal Army Medical Corps—Famous British Regiments*, Major T. H. Edwards.
The Ships of Youth, Geraldine Edge and Mary E. Johnston.
The Story of British Railways, Tatford Barrington.
1946 *History of the British Railways during the 1939–1945 War*, R. Bell.
War on the Line, Bernard Darwin.
The L.M.S. at War, G. C. Nash.
1948 *International Maritime Dictionary*, Rene de Kerchove.
The Jubilee Scrapbook of the Royal Army Medical Corps (1898–1948).
1950 *British Battles and Medals*, Major T. L. Gordon.
1951 *Not Least in the Crusade*, Peter Lovegrove.
1951 *Five Naval Journals—1798–1817. Memoirs of Peter Cullen, Esq.*
Naval Surgeon, Rear-Admiral H. G. Thursfield.
1952 *History of the Second World War—The Emergency Services*, Lieut-Colonel C. D. Dunn.
1953 *One Hundred Years of Army Nursing*, Ian Hay.
Union Castle Chronicle 1853–1953, Marischal Murray.
1954 *Photographer of the Crimean War*, Roger Fenton.
The Medical History of the Second World War—Royal Naval Medical Services, HMSO.
Voice from the Ranks, R. F. Timothy Gowring.
1956 *British Railway History—1830–1876*, Hamilton Ellis.
Battle Honours of the Royal Navy, Oliver Warner.
1957 *Boat Trains and Channel Packets*, Rixon Bucknell.
1958 *History of the Second World War—RAF Medical Services*, HMSO.
1959 *An Historical Geography of the Railways of the British Isles*, E. F. Carter.
Grey touched with Scarlet, Joan Bowden.
1960 *These Splendid Ships*, David Divine.
Wilfred Grenfell, His Life and Work, J. Lenox Kerr.
Charles Eliott, RN, Clagette Stoke.
1961 *Victorian Comfort*, John Gloag.
1962 *Europe in the Nineteenth and Twentieth Centuries—1789–1950.*
London Railways, E. Course.
World Year Book Encyclopaedia.
1963 *British Passenger Liners of the Five Oceans*, Commander C. R. Vernon Gibbs.
The Railway Lovers Companion, B. Morgan.
Railways, Loxton.
Troopships and Their History, Colonel H. C. B. Rogers.

1964 *The History of Railways*, Berghaus Erwin.
Early Railways, J. B. Snell.
History of the GWR—Vol 11, E. T. MacDermott, MA, Revised by C. R. Clinker.
The Lost Generation, Reginald POUND.
All about Ships and Shipping, Edwin P. Harnack.
1965 *A Bibliography of British Railways*, George Ottley.
Great Central, George Dow.
The London and South Western Railway, O. S. Nock.
The Story of Scapa Flow, Geoffrey Cousins.
1966 *The British Red Cross in Action*, Dame Beryl Oliver, GBE, RRC.
Salute the Soldier, Captain Eric Wheeler, RN.
1967 *Steam Railways of Britain in Colour*, O. S. Nock.
Light Railways in the First World War, W. J. K. Davies.
The Story of Passenger Transport in Britain, J. Joyce.
History of the Great Western Railway—Vol 3, O. S. Nock.
A Good Uniform—The St John Story, Joan Clifford.
Points and Signals, Michael Robbins.
Britains Railways—World War 1, J. A. B. Hamilton.
North Star to Southern Cross, John M. Maber.
1968 *The Pictorial Encyclopaedia of Railways*, Hamilton Ellis.
Railway History in Pictures—North-West England, John Patmore.
A History of the Southern Railway, C. F. Dendy Marshall.
Railway and Other Steamers, Duckworth and Langmuir.
Railways—A Readers Guide, E. F. Bryant.
The British Army in 1914, Major R. Money Bames.
The British Seaman, Christopher Lloyd.
The History of the United States, John A. Garraty.
The Rescue Ships, Vice-Admiral H. B. Schofield and Lieut-Commander L. F. Martyn.
1969 *Couplings to the Khyber*, P. S. A. Berridge.
Devon Life—Volume 5—No 39—September, Roy Faires Ltd, Exeter.
The Chanak Affair, David Walder.
1970 *Ships of the Royal Navy. An Historical Index*, J. J. Colledge.
Doctor to the Trawlermen, Dr R. W. Scott, OBE. Article in World Medicine—28 October, 1970.
The Long Carry, R. H. Haigh and P. W. Turner.
The History of the Dreadnought Seamen's Hospital at Greenwich, A. G. McBride, AHA, Seamens Hospital Management Committee, Greenwich.
1971 *The First Day of the Somme*, Martin Middlebrook.
For the Service of Mankind, Joan Clifford.
History of the Royal Army Dental Corps, Leslie J. Godden, OBE.
1972 *The Royal Army Medical Corps*, Redmond McLaughlin.
1974 *A History of the Army Medical Department*, Lt-General Sir Neil Cantlie.

Why Sink A Hospital Ship?, Dr Gordon McCulloch, Nursing Times, 18 April.

Miscellaneous

History of the Second World War.
United Kingdom Medical Services, HMSO.
The Army Medical Services Magazine, from first issue as 'The Corps Supplement—Journal of the Royal Army Medical Corps' in 1921 to the present date.
Royal Mail, 1839–1939, T. A. Bushnell.
Naval Medical History of the 1914–1918 War, Admiralty 980.
A Popular History of the Great War, Sir J. A. Hamerton.
Times History of the War, Volumes VI, VII, X, XI and XIV.
Railways in Wartime, E. F. Carter.
Railway Liveries, E. F. Carter.
British Ambulance Trains on the Continent, British Transport Historical Records.
Dunkirk and the Great Western, Ashley Brown.
Royal Army Medical Corps, Anthony Cotterell.
Records of Railway Interests in the War—Parts 1 to 17. Railway News, 91 Temple Chambers, London.
Battle of Jutland. Personal Experiences of members of the British Fleet. Maclure, Macdonald and Co. Glasgow.
Illustrated London News—volumes dated 1854, 1860, 1899 to 1901 and 1914–1915.

INDEX

Aba, 51, 57, 58
Abyssinia: Italian invasion of, 69; in Second World War, 143–4
Acadia, U.S. hospital ship, 57
Addu Atol, 60–2
Aden, 60
'Aeromedevac' scheme, 157
Agadir, 17
Aisne, Battle of (1914), 104, 107, 117
Albatross, see Miranda
Albert, fishing fleet hospital ship, 76, 79
Aldershot, Cambridge and Connaught Hospitals, 130
Alexandra, Princess of Wales (Queen Alexandra), 32
Alexandra, stern-wheel steamer, 31
Alexandria, 69
Alice Miller, fishing fleet hospital ship, 77
Alkin, Elizabeth ('Parliament Joan'), 15
Alliance, railway locomotive in Crimea, 81
Alma, Battle of, 25, 26
Alpha, fishing fleet hospital ship, 77, 78
Amarapoora, 57, 58
Ambulance Flotilla, No.1, 39
Ambulance Train Committee: First World War, 115; Second World War, 138, 139
Ambulance Train Depots and Supply Stores: Abbeville, 115; Arquata, 118
Ambulance Transports, 34, 35
American Civil War, 83–5; special hospital trains, 85, 90
American Ladies in London, Committee of, 32, 67
American War of 1814, 16
Amsterdam, sunk by mine, 57
Andes, 25
Anglia, mined, 42–3
Anne, Queen, 14
Anzio landings (1944), 56, 60
Aquitania, 38, 39, 129, 131
Arabi revolt (1882), 30
Arcadian, casualty station ship for Oran, 57
Archangel, 49, 144
Argon, army hospital carrier, 18
Argonaut, HMS. base hospital, Chatham, 16
Army Dental Corps, 51
Army Hospital Corps, 27, 28
Army Nursing Service, 82
Arrogant, HMS, 137
Ashanti Wars, 16
Asia, 22
Assam, 42
Asturias, 35–6, 103; naval hospital ship, 36; handed over to army, 36; torpedoed, 36, 44, 46; rebuilt as cruising liner *Arcadian*, 36
Atlantis, 51, 54

Australia, 122; Army Medical Services, 48; medical personnel in Britain, 129
Austrian Maltese Order, 88
Austrian system, 89
Austro-Hungarian Red Cross Society, 90
Austro-Prussian-Italian War (1866), 82–3, 85–6
Avon, 26

Baghdad Railway, 120
Baker, Bernard H., 67
Balaklava, railway works, 81, 82
Balentia, 17
Balkan Wars (1912–13), 33, 83
Barnton Tramway system, 117
Base hospitals, 16–17
'Bath-train' in Romania, 121
Bay State, U.S. hospital ship, 31
Belgian Government Mail Steamers, 37
Belgian refugees in First World War, 161
Belle of Dunkerque, 30
Belleisle, 73
Bien Charge, Le, 15
Berlin system, 89
Birmingham Carriage and Railway Wagon Company, 94, 106, 112
Boer rebellion (1881), 83
Boer War (1899–1902), *see* South African War
Bombay, wooden paddle steamer, 26
Boulomie system, 89
Boxer Rebellion (1900), 33, 67
Braemar Castle, 48–9; mined, 43–4
Bréchot-Déspres-Amelines stretcher-carrying system, 89, 98–102, 119, 120, 128
Bridport, Lord, 16
Brighton, 146; sunk in air raid, 51
Britannia, Royal Yacht, designed for adaptation as hospital ship, 159
Britannic, 39, 129; mined, 43

British Ambulance Trains:
 First World War; Nos. 1, 2, and 3, 101–3; Nos. 5–7, 103; No. 8, 104; Nos. 9 and 10, 105; No. 11, 106, 113; No. 12 ('Khaki' train), 111–12; No. 14 ('Queen Mary's' train), 112; No. 15 ('Princess Christian' train), 112–13; Nos. 16 and 17, 113; No. 18, 118; Nos. 19 and 20, 113; No. 21, 118; No. 23, 114; No. 24, 118; Nos. 25–38, 113, 118; No. 39, 113–15, 118; No. 40, 120; No. 41, 113, 115, 118; No. 42, 113, 115; No. 43, 113, 115, 118; Nos. 44–51, 120; Nos. 52 and 53, 120; Nos. 56 and 57, 120; Nos. 61 and 62, 129
 Second World War; No. 3, 145; No. 4, 146–7; No. 6, 147–8; No. 13, 144–5; No. 63, 141, 142
British Army of the Rhine (BAOR), ambulance trains since 1950, 156–8; conversion of German passenger coaches, 156; disbandment of RAMC staff, 157; use for RAMC (TAVR) training, 157, 158; composition of trains, 157–8
British Pacific Fleet, 59, 66, 69
British Red Cross Society, 29–32, 40, 41, 48, 88, 106, 123, 160–2; Scottish Branch, 17; and Army Medical Services, 31, 91; Joint War Committee with Order of St John, 113, 121, 141; war organization (1939–45), 139; provision of comforts and amenities, 160–2
Burke, Anna, 31
Burma, operations in Second World War, 59, 65, 143
Bury, rescue ship, 64

Caledonia, HMS, *see Dreadnought*
Caledonian Railway, 114, 136
Cambria, 25
Cameroons, the, 42, 121

Canada, 122; Army Medical Service tramcars, 116; medical personnel in Britain, 129
Canterbury and Whitstable Railway, 80
Cap St Jacques, French vessel, 62
Cartagena, expedition to (1714), 21
Carthage, 30
Casualty Evacuation Trains Committee (1938) 149
Catania, Duke of Sutherland's steam yacht, 37
Cecelia, 17
Central Medical War Committee Second World War, 154
'Chanak Affair' (1922), 123
Chancellorsville, Battle of, 84
Charles II, 14, 21
Charon, 16
Chatham, 16; naval ambulance train at, 135–7
China, HMHS, 17, 19
China Wars: (1839–42), 16; (1860), 28–9; construction and equipment of hospital ships, 28–9
Cholera, 26, 72, 73
Churchill, Lady Randolph, 32, 67
Churchill, (Sir) Winston, 67
City of Athens, 42
Civil Nursing Reserve, 154–5
Clacton, mine-sweeper, 48
Classic, HMHS, 17, 19
'Collis dandy' apparatus, 88
Cologne Express, 123
Colombo, 60–2
Compt de Beaufort system, 89
Coromandel, HMS, 16
Corps of Hospital Orderlies, 27, 28
Cosham, Alexandra Hospital, 130
Courland, 30
Crane, trawler, 78
Crimean War, 16, 25–8, 160; hospitals at Scutari, 25–7; cholera, 26; personnel of hospital ships, 27–8; numbers of sick and wounded carried, 28; railways, 81–2

Cromwell, Oliver, 21
Cross-channel steamers as hospital ships, 35
D-Day, *see* Normandy landings
Daffodil, at Zeebrugge, 137
Dardanelles campaign, 18, 38, 39, 41, 47–8, 129, 131; 'black' and 'white' ships, 48; list of hospital ships, etc, used for casualties, 169
Deal, temporary hospital, 15
Decauville system, 116, 120
Deep sea fishermen, hospital ships for, 73–9
De Forest, Dr, 121
Devonshire, 73
Diary of a Nursing Sister on the Western Front, 1914–15 (Luard), 108
Dinard, 52, 56; mined, 57
Dispensaries on hospital ships, 29
Dogger Bank, 75; 'Incident' (1904), 78
Donegal, torpedoed, 45
Dongola, 47
Donna, see Miranda
Donovan, Surgeon-General W. (Sir William), 125–6
Dover: reception port in First World War, 127–8, 131–2, 137; Marine Station, 128
Dover, HMS, 73
Dover Castle, torpedoed, 45
Dreadnought, name of two hospital ships for merchant seamen, 73
Dreadnought Seamen's Hospital Greenwich, 73, 136
Drina, HMHS, 17
Dunant, Jean Henri, 35
Dunbar, sailing ship, 26
Dunkirk, evacuation from (1940), 51–4, 140
Dunluce Castle, 42
Durban, 61, 62, 67

East Africa in First World War, 42, 121

Eastern Fleet (Second World War), 59, 61, 62
Ebani, 42
Edge Geraldine, 55
Edward VII, King, 75
Egypt: campaigns in, 30–2, 83, 160; in First World War, 119–20
Egypt, 32, 37
Egyptian Red Crescent Society, 119
El Nil, 63
Elliot, Commander Charles, 16
Embarkation Medical Service, 125–6
Empire Clyde, see Maine
Empress of India, see Loyalty
Ensign, fishing fleet hospital ship, 74
Entente Cordiale ('Franco-British') train, 102–3
Exmouth, Lord, 73

Falmouth, proposal for hospital at, 23–4
Fieldhouse, W. J., 94, 106, 112
First World War, 17–20, 34–50 78, 89, 161–2
  military hospital ships, 35–7; giant liners as hospital ships, 38–40; ward barges, 39–40; ward barges, 39–40; hospital ships torpedoed and mined, 42–6; Gallipoli campaign, 18, 38, 39, 41, 47–8, 129, 131, 169; list of military hospital ships, etc, 166–8
  military ambulance trains overseas, 98–124; French *trains sanitaires*, 98–9, 101; British ambulance train service, 101–2; *Entente Cordiale train*, 102–3; battles in 1914, 103–4, 103–4; specially constructed trains, 111–13; standard pattern trains, 113, 115; depot and supply stores, 115; temporary trains, 116; 'trench railways', 116; number of patients carried, 117–18, 124; Italy, 118–19; Egypt, 119–20; Salonika, 120; Africa, 121–2; U.S. trains, 122–3, 181–4; growth of service in France, 175–6; capacity of trains in France, Sept 1915, 177
  military ambulance trains in U.K. 125–32, 185; trains from railway companies, 126–7; trains from Irish railways, 126–7; Dover and Southampton, 127–8; number of trains, 128; distribution of patients on arrival, 129–30; military hospitals, 130–1; general hospitals mobilized, 131; statistics, 131–2
  naval ambulance trains in U.K., 133–7; moveable cot system, 133–4; No. 1 Train, 135, 136, 187–8; No. 2 Train, 135; No. 3 Train, 135, 137; No. 4 Train, 135; No. 5 Train, 135, 137; operations and routes, 135–6; types of train, 136; Battle of Jutland, 136–7; Zeebrugge operations, 136, 137
Flûte hôpital, 15
Flûte Royale, La, 15
Flying Kestrel, sea-going tug, 19–20
Forrester, Lt-Col F.S., 95
Fortune, La, 15
France: hospital ships, 13, 21 use of 'railway sick transport carriage', 82; *Chemin de Fer de l'Ouest*, 86; *trains sanitaires*, 98–9, 101; French offer of trains for British forces, 140; British trains in France (1939–40), 140
Franconia, torpedoed and sunk, 41
Franco-Prussian War, 83, 94; Prussian system for evacuation of sick and wounded, 87
Friends Ambulance Unit, 113
Furley, Sir John, 94, 96, 106, 112
Future: of military ambulance trains, 158–9; of hospital ships, 159

Galeka, hospital carrier, 18
Galician, see Glenhart Castle

Gallipoli, *see* Dardanelles Campaign
Ganges, steel-hulled ship, 30, 31
Garth Castle, 17
Gascon, 42
Gauvin spring stretcher, 86
Geddes, Elizabeth, 31
Geneva, conference in, 35
Geneva Convention, 34, 35, 42, 55, 63
George V, King, 105
German, 32, 95; renamed *Glengorm Castle*, 37
German prisoners of war in Britain, 129
German Red Cross Society, 97
German South-West Africa, operations against, 42
Gerusalemme, Italian passenger liner, 62
Gettysburg, Battle of, 84
Gibson, Isabella, 31
Glengorm Castle, see *German*
Glenart Castle, 37; mined, 44
'Glorious First of June', 16
Gloucester Castle, torpedoed, 44, 45
Goodwill, first recorded English hospital ship, 13
Goorkha, mined, 46
Gordon, Lt-Col J. H., 24
Gorgon, HMS, 16
Grampus, hospital ship for merchant seamen, 72–3
Grand Saint-Augustin, Le, 15
Great Central Railway, 126–8
Great Eastern Railway, 126, 127
Great Indian Peninsular Railway, 122
Great Southern and Western Railway (Ireland), 127
Great Tasmania, 27–8
Great War, *see* First World War
Great Western Railway, 126, 127, 138, 139, 151, 153
Great Western Railway (Ireland), 126, 127
Greenwich Hospital, 72, 73

Grenfell, (Sir) Wilfred Thomason, 75–8; Grenfell Associations, 78
Grianaig, 19
'Gripe' suspension system, 134
Gripsholm, 57
Grund system, 87, 89
Guildford Castle, 17, 42, 46
Gunships, converted to hospital ships, 15
Gurley system, 89
Gurlt, Dr, and *paillasse* method, 83–4, 86
Gwalior, 33
Gwalior, Maharajah of, 37

Hague, The, conferences at, 35
Haifa-Damascus railway, 120
Hall, Inspector-General John, 25–6
Hamburg system, 89
Hardinge, 33
Harmonic, collier, 20
Haslar, Royal Naval Hospital, 72
Heidelberg system, 89
Heliopolis, see *Maine*
Herring, 22
HMLST 363, 65
Hong Kong, 62, 70
Hôpital de l'armée, 15
Hopwood, Francis (Lord Southborough), 75
Hospital carriers, 34
Hospital Conveyance Corps, 82
Hospital drifters, 66
Hospital tenders, 66
Huskisson, William, 81
Hythe, mine-sweeper, 48

Icelandic 'Cod War', 79
Illumination of hospital ships and carriers, 34
India, 120, 122; repatriation of invalids from, 29; ports used in Second World War, 60–2; carriage of patients in railway vehicles, 88–9; ambulance trains produced in Second World War, 143
Inkerman, Battle of, 28

197

International Grenfell Association, 78–9
Iphigenia, 73
Ireland: railways supply ambulance trains in First World War, 126–7; military hospitals, 131
Iris, at Zeebrugge, 137
Isle of Jersey, HMHS, 52, 53, 57, 58
Italian-Austrian War (1859), 82, 83
Italy: ambulance trains in First World War, 118–19; State Railways, 119; Maltese Order, 119; in Second World War, 144

Jamaica, 24; hospital ships proposed for, 23
James II, King, 14
Jan Breydel, 37
Jean, 22
Johnston, Mary, 55
Joseph and Sarah Miles, fishing fleet hospital ship, 77, 78
Journal of the Royal Army Medical Corps, 107
Jutland, Battle of, 19, 136–7

Kalyan, 49
Kangaroo, steamship, 26
Karapara, HMHS, 17, 19, 36, 45, 62
Karoa, 62
Keate, Surgeon-General T., report on hospital ships, 22–4
Knights of Malta and the Grand Priory of Bohemia, hospital train, 89–90
Konigin Regentes, Dutch hospital ship, 46
Korean War (1950–53), 70–1

Labrador fishermen and fisheries, 74–9; 'Liveyers', 76
Lady Juliana, 23
Ladysmith, siege of, 95
Lancashire and Yorkshire Railway, 126–8
Land Transport Corps, 82
Landing Ships Infantry, 65

Landing ships Tank (LST), 65
Lanfranc, torpedoed, 45
Laundresses, 14, 15
Laurie, Major-General, 88
Leake, 14
Le Conte, Pierre, 15
Leinster, 54–6
Leonardo da Vinci, see *Maine*
Leslie, Major R. W. D., 128
Liberty, 19
Lileham, 31
Liners as hospital ships, 17, 37–40
Linxweiler system, 89, 120
Liverpool and Manchester Railway, 80
Llandovery Castle: (1918) torpedoed, 46; (1942), 54
Locomotion, Stephenson's engine, 80
London and North Eastern Railway, 138, 139, 151, 153
London and North Western Railway, 125–7, 129
London and South Western Railway, 97, 126–9, 135, 151
London Belle, 49
London Hospital, The, 74
London Midland and Scottish Railway, 138, 139, 151, 153
London Scottish Regiment, 101–8
Longmoor Military Railway, 140, 157
Longmore, Surgeon-General Sir T., 90
Loos, Battle of, 117–18
Lowe, P., 95
Loyalty (former *Empress of India*), 37, 38
Luard, Sister K. E., 108–11
Lusitania, collier, 43

Macedonia, 120
Mackay, Staff Sgt. Angus, 26
Macpherson, Major W. D. (Major-Gen. Sir William), 97
Madagascar Campaign (1942), 54

198

Magnificent, hospital and store ship, 16
Maid of Kent, 146; bombed and sunk, 51–2
Maine, HMHS: first ship, 20, 31–3, 67; second ship (former *Swansea*), 68; third ship (former *Heliopolis*), 68; fourth ship (former *Panama*), 58, 68–9; fifth ship (former *Empire Clyde*, *Leonardo da Vinci*), 69–71, 159
Malaya, reoccupation of, 62
Malcolm, HMS, 16
Malta, 68, 69
Manual of the Medical Staff Corps (1893), 89
Marconi, Guglielmo, 77
Mariner's Journal, The, 15
Mariner's Mirror, The, 13
Markings of hospital ships and carriers, 34
Martha, 14
Mather, E. J., 74
Mauretania, 39, 40, 129
Mauritius, sail-rigged steam ship, 28
Mayflower, 31
Medical History of the Second World War-Royal Naval Medical Services, 57
Medical Staff Corps, 28
Melbourne, sail-rigged steam ship, 28
Memory in Solferino, A (Dunant), 35
Merchant seamen, hospital ships for, 72–3
Mercia, 26
Mesopotamia, 40–1, 121
Michelham, Lord and Lady, 112
Michelin Diesel Auto-Rail cars, 144
Midland Railway, 126, 127
Midnight Sun, see Princess of Wales
Military hospitals, 130–1
Millbank, Queen Alexandra Military Hospital, 130
Mina, trawler, 78
Minden, HMS, 16

Mine-sweepers used for evacuating casualties, 48
Miranda (formerly *Albatross*, *Donna*), fishing fleet hospital ship, 79
Mississippi River, 'floating hospital' on, 29
Missouri, U.S. hospital ship, 31
Mobile Railway, 85
Mombasa–Nairobi Railway, 121
Mons, retreat from (1914), 102
Moore, Major G. A., 107–8
Morache system, 89
Motor Fishing Vessels (MFVs), 66
Motor-launches, 40–1, 48
Moulmein, trawler, 78
Mundy, Baron, 86, 88
Murmansk, 48–9, 121, 144

Nahba, river hospital ship, 41
National Aid Society, Princess of Wales Branch, 160
National Health Society, 74
National Mission to Deep Sea Fishermen (Royal), 74–5, 77–9
National Society for Aid to Sick and Wounded, 31
Naval hospital ships, 1608–1740, list, 163–4
Netherlands South African Railway, Pretoria, 97
Netley, Royal Victoria Hospital, 29, 97, 120, 130; Museum of Military Surgery, 86; carriage to transport patients from Portsmouth, 90; 'Netley Coaches' 96–7, 126, 139, 186; handed over to USA in Second World War, 139–40
Neuve Chapelle, Battle of (1915), 117
New Zealand: Army Medical Services, 48; medical personnel in Britain, 129
Newfoundland, 55; sunk by aircraft, 55–6, 58
Newfoundland fishermen and fisheries, 74–9
Newhaven, No. 1 Ambulance Port for BEF, 52, 54

199

Newmarket, mine-sweeper, 48
Niger, 23
Nightingale, Florence, 82, 160
Normandy landings (1944), 57, 58, 65, 141, 142, 162
North Africa, Allied invasion (1942), 59, 66
North British Railway, 135, 136
North Eastern Railway vans, 127
North German Confederation, plan for rail conveyance of severely wounded, 87
North Sea fishermen, 73–5, 77, 78
Northumbrian, locomotive, 81
North-West Africa, in Second World War, 144
Norwegian campaign (1940), 51, 58
Nubia, 33

Ophir: First World War, 17; Dutch vessel requisitioned in Second World War, 61–2
Orcana, 32
Orford, 15
Orient, 27
Orsino, fishing fleet hospital ship, 79
Osmanieh, 30, 160
Ossory, 15
Oxfordshire: (HMHS No. 1), 17, 36; Second World War, 57, 59–60

P & O and B. I. Lines, 37
Pacific Fleet Train, 60
Paillasse method, 83–4
Palestine troubles (1936), 69
Panama, 20
 see also *Maine*
Paris, bombed and sunk, 51
Paris *Exposition Internationale* (1867), experiments on carriage of sick and wounded, 86, 87
Paul Paix, 19
Peninsular War, 24–5
Pharon, HMS, 16
Philadelphia Railroad Company, 84–5
Pieter de Connick, 37

Plassy, HMHS, 17, 19
PLM Railway Company, 105
Ponts system, 89
Portugal, Russian hospital ship, 46
Pride of the Ocean, converted into hulk for patients, 27
Princess, steam launch, 31
Princess Christian Hospital Trains: first train; in South Africa, 32, 93–6, 112, 173; in South-West Africa in First World War, 121–2; second train; in First World War, 112–13; coaches in Turkey (1922), 123
Princess May, steam launch, 76
Princess of Wales (former yachting cruiser *Midnight Sun*), 32–3
Princess Royal, HMS, 19
Prisoners of war: enemy prisoners in British Isles, 129, 132; repatriated British prisoners (1944), 141
Prussian Commissions on rail transport for sick and wounded, 86, 87

Queen Alexandra, fishing fleet hospital ship, 77
Queen Mary's Ambulance Train, 112
Queen Victoria: fishing fleet hospital ship, 77; steam launch, 30–1
Quetta earthquake (1935), 123–4

Rachid, ex-Egyptian customs vessel, 41
Railway Companies Ambulance Centres, 161
Railway Executive Committee, 138, 149
Railway Groups (1938–39), 138, 149
Red Cross Societies, International Congresses, 87, 97
Redbreast, mine-sweeper, 48
Relief, U.S. hospital ship, 31
Rescue Ships accompanying convoys, 63–4

Rescue Ships, The (Schofield and Martyn), 64
Rewa, HMHS, 17–19; torpedoed, 18–19
Rhodesia, rebellion in (1896), 83
Robert Sale, 27
Rocket, Joshua, 24
Rocket, Stephenson's locomotive, 81
Roebuck, 52
Romania, 121
Rome Red Cross Special Ambulance Train, 119
Ross, Lt. N. H., 31
Royal Army Medical Corps, 28, 31, 43, 44, 46, 55, 101–2, 157; *Journal*, 107; Territorial Force, 131; TAVR, 157, 158
Royal Army Medical Corps Training (1911), 89, 109
Royal Corps of Transport, 79; Railway Squadron, 157
Royal Engineers, No. 1 Workshop Company, 139
Royal Navy, list of Hospital Ships on service with, 1790–1854, 165
Russia: in First World War, 121; Servian divisions in, 121; allied intervention in North Russia, 48–9, 132; trains between Murmansk and Archangel in Second World War, 144
Russo-Japanese War, 33, 78, 83, 160
Russo-Turkish War, 30, 88

Sadowa, Battle of, 85
Sailors' wives in hospital ships, 14
St Andrew, 35, 52, 55–7, 128
St Andrew's Ambulance Association, 161
St David, 35, 52, 56–7
St Helier, 52
St Hilda, 27
Saint-Jacques de Portugal, Le, 15
St John of Jerusalem, Order of, 113, 121, 141, 161; Ambulance Brigade, 74, 94n, 95, 154

St Julien, 52, 53, 56
St Margaret of Scotland, 17
St Patrick, 35
Saladin, 27
Salerno landings (1943), 55–6, 58
Salonika, 118, 120
Salta, 17, 36; mined, 44
Savory and Moore's 'patent safeguard bottles', 29
Scapa Flow, 19, 58, 66, 78
Schleswig-Holstein War (1864), 82
Schofield, A., 74
Seamen's Hospital Society, 72–3
Second World War, 51–66, 162; Norwegian campaign, 51, 58; evacuation from Dunkirk, 51–4, 140; activities in Mediterranean, 54–9, 62, 66, 69; Normandy landings, 57, 58, 65, 141, 142; Royal Naval Hospital Ships, 58–63; war against Japan, 59–62; Rescue Ships, 63–4; Landing Ships Infantry and Tank, 65; Motor Fishing Vessels, 66; list of Hospital Ships etc, 170–1

military ambulance trains, 138–48; composition of trains, 139; trains for U.S. forces, 139–40; British trains in France (1939–40); 140, 144–8; statistics, 141; casualties after D-Day, 141; Burma, 143; East Africa, 143–4; North-West Africa, 144

naval casualties, 141–3; coaches converted for naval transport, 142–3; admissions of patients to naval hospital ships, 172

casualty evacuation trains in U.K, 149–55; plans before war, 149–50; Train No. 53, 150; improvised ambulance trains, 150; trains reserved for civilians, 150–1; Train No. 33, 151; carriage of civilian patients from danger areas, 151; transport of service sick and wounded, 151;

Second World War—(cont)
little used for air raid casualties, 151; release of many trains, 152; composition and accommodation, 152–3; staffing, 153–4; equipment, 154; principal movements of trains, 154–5; statistics, 154–5
Seminole, U.S. hospital ship, 57
Seraphis, convalescent ship, 16
Servian-Bulgarian War (1885–86) 83, 88
Servian Divisions in Russia, First World War, 121
Shamrock, U.S. hospital ship, 57
Shanking, 42
Ships of Youth, The, (Edge and Johnston), 55
Shrivenham, reception of U.S. casualties at, 139
Sicily, invasion of, 54, 59
Sick and Wounded (Sick and Hurt) Board, 15
Simon, HMS, 16
Sinai Peninsula, 119
Singapore, 61, 62
Smith, Andrew, 25
Société Française, Sanitary Train, 89
Societies for Aid to Wounded in Time of War, 86
Solace, U.S. hospital ship, 31
Somali, 17, 18
Somaliland: operations (1903–4), 33; in Second World War, 143–4
Somersetshire, 54
Somme, first battle of (1916), 40, 118, 132; statistics of evacuation of casualties, 178–80
Soudan, HMHS, 17: Dardanelles campaign, 18
South Africa: Medical Corps, 42; Red Cross Society, 42; Railways, 122
South African War (1899–1902); 31–3, 37, 67, 68, 83, 126, 160–1; military hospital trains, 90–8; conversion of ordinary trains, 91; categories of trains, 91–2; composition of trains, 92–3; Princess Christian Hospital Train, 32, 93–6, 112, 173; No. 4 Hospital Train, 96–7, 174; Boer hospital trains, 97; 'Netley Coaches', 96–7
South East Asia Command, 66
South Eastern and Chatham Railway, 127, 135
South-West Africa in First World War, 95, 121–2
Southampton: reception port in First World War, 127–8, 131, 132, 161; in Second World War, 141
Southern Railway, 138, 150, 151, 153
Spanish-American War (1898), 31
Spanish Armada, 13
Spanish Civil War, 69
Spartan, 31–2
Stad Antwerpen, 37
Stella, yacht, 31, 160
Stephenson, George, 80, 81
Stewart, Dr E., 96, 97
Stockport, rescue ship, 64
Stockton and Darlington Railway, 80
Strathcona and *Strathcona II*, fishing fleet hospital ships, 77–8
Strathcona, Lord, 77
Suakin expedition (1885), 30
Sudan expedition (1898), 31, 33
Supple, Colonel J. F., 91
Surgeries in hospital ships, 29
Sutherland, Duke of, 37
Sutherland, J. J., 13, 15
Swansea, see Maine
Sweden, 122
Swindon, U.S. ambulance train maintenance unit at, 139
Sydney, 27
Sylvester, Assistant Surgeon Henry, 26

Tairea, 55, 62
Talamba, bombed and sunk, 57, 62
Tanda, P. and O. liner, 37

Tangier, evacuation of (1683), 21
Tebbut, Misses, 161
Thames Church Mission, 74
Thomson, Assistant Surgeon James, 26
Tice, Staff Surgeon Major, 26
Tigris, River, 40–1
Tjitjalengka, Dutch vessel, 61
Tobruk, 54, 60
Togoland, 121
Torbay Review (1910), 67
Tournelle, HMS, hospital hulk, 16
'Trench railways', 116
Trent, 27
'Trestle' stretcher-carrying system, 128–9
Treves, (Sir) Frederick, 75
Trincomalee, 61, 62
Trojan, 31–2
Turco-Greek War (1897), 83
Turco-Servian War (1876), 29–30

United States: Seventh Fleet 60; 'U.S.A.' trains, 122–3, 181–4; trains for forces in U.K., Second World War, 139–40
Unity, 21
Unknown Warriors (Luard), 111

V.A.D.'s, 161
Vasna, HMHS, 58–9
Ventilation in hospital ships, 22–3, 29
Vestibule vans, 129
Victor Emanuel, HMS, 16
Victoria, Queen, 160
Victory, railway locomotive in Crimea, 81
Ville de Liège, 37
Vindictive, HMS, 137

Vita, 57, 60–1
Von Roon, Prussian War Minister, 83
Vpered, Russian hospital ship, 46

Walcheren expedition, 24
Walton Belle, 49
War Department Ambulance Trains ('Netley Coaches'), 97, 126–8, 130, 139, 157, 186
War Railway Council, 125
Ward barges, 39–40
Warilda, torpedoed, 46
Waterhen, HMAS, 60
Waterloo, Battle of, 25
Welcome, 21
West Africa campaign (1895), 16
West Indies, bringing invalids home from, 23–4
Willemstad, withdrawal from (1749), 22
William Jackson, 27
Wilson, Surgeon-General Sir W. D., 96
Wishart, Assistant Surgeon James, 26
Woolwich, Royal Herbert Hospital, 130
Wu Sueh, 62

Yachts as hospital ships, 19, 37
Young, J. S., 30
Ypres: Battle of (1914), 103–4; Second Battle of (1915), 117
Yusef Kamel, Prince, 119

Zavodovski stretcher-carrying system, 88, 89, 120, 122, 128
Zeebrugge operations (1918) 136, 137
Zulu War (1879), 83, 160

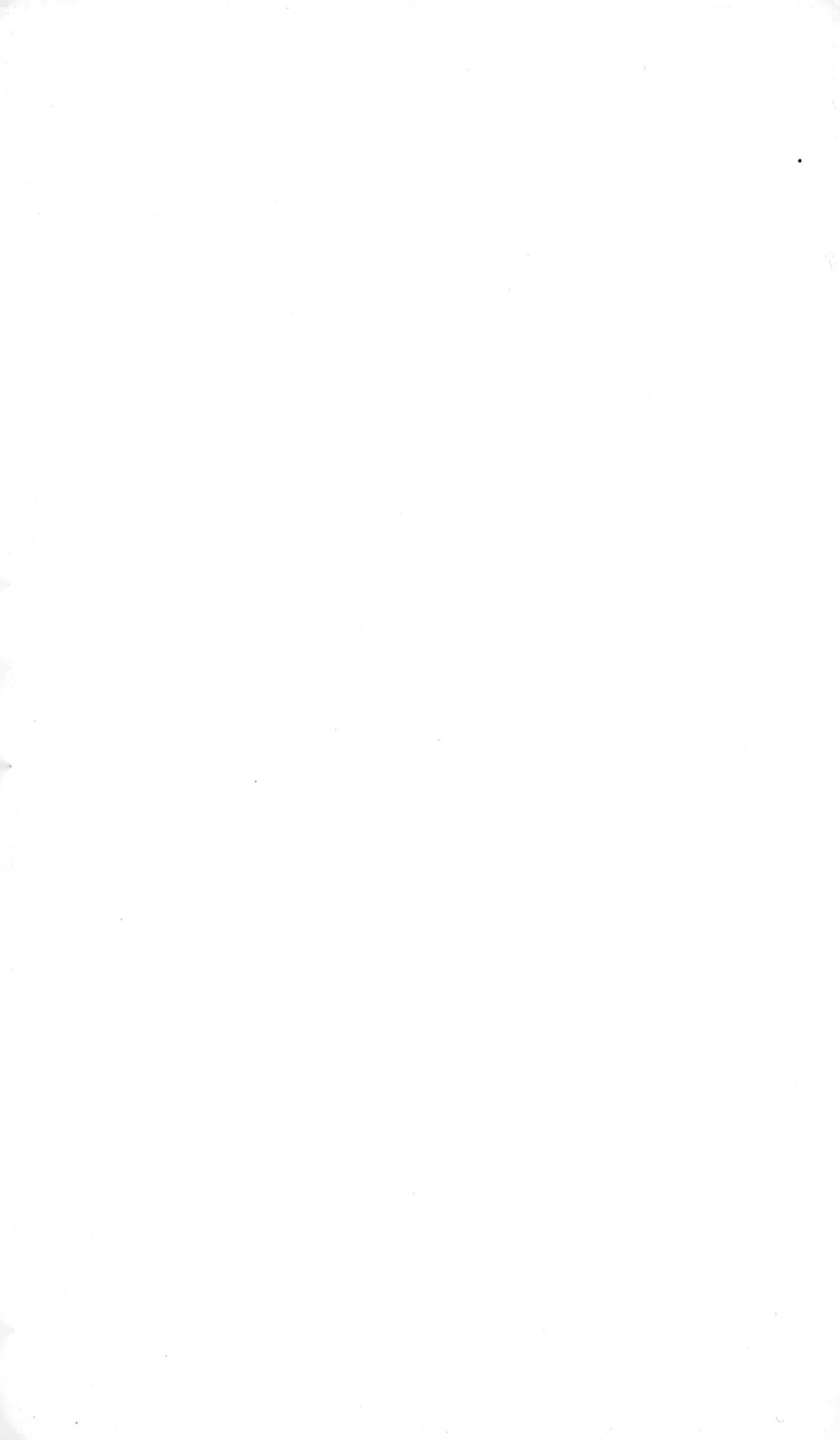